Understanding
Clinical
Research

Understanding Clinical Research

Editors

Renato D. Lopes, MD, MHS, PhD
Executive Director, Brazilian Clinical Research Institute
Federal University of São Paulo, São Paulo, Brazil
Associate Professor of Medicine, Division of Cardiology
Department of Medicine, Duke University Medical Center
Associate Program Director, Fellowship Program
Duke Clinical Research Institute
Durham, North Carolina

Robert A. Harrington, MD
Chair, Department of Medicine
Stanford University
Stanford, California

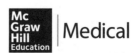 Medical

New York   Chicago   San Francisco   Lisbon   London   Madrid   Mexico City
Milan   New Delhi   San Juan   Seoul   Singapore   Sydney   Toronto

Understanding Clinical Research

Drs. Lopes and Harrington receive no royalties from the sales of this book. In addition, they donate their portion of the sales proceeds to the Duke Clinical Research Institute's Fellowship Program, to enhance the education and support of future generations of clinical researchers

1 2 3 4 5 6 7 8 9 0   DOC/DOC   18 17 16 15 14 13

ISBN 978-0-07-174678-6
MHID 0-07-174678-1

This book was set in Minion by Aptara, Inc.
The editors were Christine Diedrich and Peter J. Boyle.
The production supervisor was Sherri Souffrance.
Project management was provided by Indu Jawwad, Aptara, Inc.
The designer was Alan Barnett.
RR Donnelley was printer and binder.

This book was printed on acid-free paper.

Library of Congress Cataloging-in-Publication Data

Understanding clinical research / editors, Renato D. Lopes, Robert A. Harrington.
   p. ; cm.
  Includes bibliographical references and index.
  ISBN 978-0-07-174678-6—ISBN 0-07-174678-1
  I. Lopes, Renato D.   II. Harrington, Robert A.
  [DNLM: 1. Biomedical Research.   2. Clinical Trials as Topic.   3. Research Design.
W 20.5]

610.72′4—dc23

                                              2012051271

McGraw-Hill Education books are available at special quantity discounts to use as premiums and sales promotions, or for use in corporate training programs. To contact a representative please e-mail us at bulksales@mcgraw-hill.com.

Contents

SECTION I: EVOLUTION OF CLINICAL RESEARCH
Renato D. Lopes, editor

Contributors

Daniel K. Benjamin Jr., MD, PhD
Professor of Pediatrics
Duke University School of Medicine
Faculty Associate Director
Duke Clinical Research Institute
Durham, North Carolina
Chapter 1

Lisa G. Berdan, MHS, PA-C
Associate Director, Cardiovascular
  Megatrials
Duke Clinical Research Institute
Durham, North Carolina
Chapter 3

Robert Bigelow, PhD
Associate Director
Duke Clinical Research Institute
Durham, North Carolina
Chapter 5

Catherine Bodine, RN
Clinical Research Communications
  Specialist III
Duke Clinical Research Institute
Durham, North Carolina
Chapter 1

Anjan K. Chakrabarti, MD
Clinical Fellow in Medicine
Department of Medicine
Division of Cardiology
Beth Israel Deaconess Medical Center
Boston, Massachusetts
Chapter 2

Karen Chiswell, PhD
Senior Biostatistician
Duke Clinical Research Institute
Durham, North Carolina
Chapters 6 and 7

**Michael Cohen-Wolkowiez, MD,
PhD**
Assistant Professor
Department of Pediatrics
Division of Infectious Disease
Duke Clinical Research Institute
Durham, North Carolina
Chapter 6

Lesley H. Curtis, PhD
Associate Professor in Medicine
Division of General Medicine
Department of Medicine
Duke University Medical Center
Durham, North Carolina

Kate Davis, RN
Clinical Research Communications
    Specialist III
Duke Clinical Research Institute
Durham, North Carolina
Chapter 1

Michaela A. Dinan, PhD
Biostatistician III, Clinical and
    Genetic Economics
Duke Clinical Research Institute
Durham, North Carolina
Chapter 10

Zubin J. Eapen, MD
Assistant Professor of Medicine
Division of Cardiology
Department of Medicine
Duke University Medical Center
Duke Clinical Research Institute
Durham, North Carolina
Chapter 16

C. Michael Gibson, MS, MD
Associate Professor of Medicine
Department of Medicine
Division of Cardiology
Beth Israel Deaconess Medical Center
Boston, Massachusetts
Chapter 2

Jeffrey T. Guptill, MD, MA
Medical Instructor
Division of Neurology
Department of Medicine
Duke University School of Medicine
Duke Clinical Research Institute
Durham, North Carolina
Chapter 7

Gail E. Hafley, MS
Senior Statistician
Duke Clinical Research Institute
Durham, North Carolina
Chapter 8

Bradley G. Hammill, MS
Senior Biostatistician, Clinical and
    Genetic Economics
Duke Clinical Research Institute
Durham, North Carolina
Chapter 12

Robert A. Harrington, MD
Chair, Department of Medicine
Stanford University
Stanford, California

Sergio Leonardi, MD
Research Scholar
Duke Clinical Research Institute
Durham, North Carolina
Chapter 8

Renato D. Lopes, MD, MHS, PhD
Executive Director, Brazilian Clinical
    Research Institute
Federal University of São Paulo
São Paulo, Brazil
Associate Professor of Medicine
Division of Cardiology
Department of Medicine
Duke University Medical Center
Associate Program Director,
    Fellowship Program
Duke Clinical Research Institute
Durham, North Carolina
Chapter 3

Karen S. Pieper, MS
Associate Director, Biostatistics
Duke Clinical Research Institute
Durham, North Carolina
Chapter 8

Craig J. Reist, PhD
Clinical Trials Project Leader III
Duke Clinical Research Institute
Durham, North Carolina
Chapter 3

Eric M. Reyes, PhD
Duke University Medical Center
Duke Clinical Research Institute
Durham, North Carolina
Chapter 15

Tyrus L. Rorick, RN
Clinical Trials Project Leader III
Duke Clinical Research Institute
Durham, North Carolina
Chapter 3

Kevin A. Schulman, MD
Professor of Medicine and Gregory
    Mario and Jeremy Mario Professor
    of Business Administration
Duke University
Associate Director, Health Services
    Research
Duke Clinical Research Institute
Durham, North Carolina
Chapter 4

Phillip J. Schulte, PhD
Duke University Medical Center
Duke Clinical Research Institute
Durham, North Carolina
Chapter 14

P. Brian Smith, MD, MHS, MPH
Chief, Division of Quantitative
    Sciences
Department of Pediatrics
Duke University Medical Center
Duke Clinical Research Institute
Durham, North Carolina
Chapter 9

Laine E. Thomas, PhD
Assistant Professor
Department of Biostatistics and
    Bioinformatics
Duke University School of Medicine
Durham, North Carolina
Chapters 14 and 15

Nidhi Tripathi, BS
Medical Student
Duke University School of Medicine
Durham, North Carolina
Chapter 1

Kevin N. Turner, MD
Clinical Fellow
Department of Pediatrics
University of North Carolina Medical
    Center
Chapel Hill, North Carolina
Chapter 9

David M. Vock, PhD
Division of Biostatistics
University of Minnesota School of
    Public Health
Minneapolis, Minnesota
Chapter 13

Kevin M. Watt, MD
Assistant Professor
Department of Pediatrics
Division of Critical Care Medicine
Duke University Medical Center
Duke Clinical Research Institute
Durham, North Carolina
Chapter 6

Yee Weng Wong, MBBS, FRACP
Research Scholar
Duke Clinical Research Institute
Durham, North Carolina
Chapter 4

Ying Xian, MD, PhD
Research Scholar
Duke Clinical Research Institute
Durham, North Carolina
Chapter 11

Foreword

Every physician is challenged to provide the very best care to patients, basing practice on the evidence generated from clinical research combined with judgment. For this to happen, two elements must be in place. First, high-quality evidence must be available and second, clinicians must know the conclusions or have access to decision support that enables translation of research into actions based on proper interpretation of the findings. Unfortunately, in many areas of medicine, large gaps exist. Clearly, more and higher-quality studies are desperately needed to address the major unanswered questions in clinical practice. But perhaps equally important is the need to empower clinicians to appreciate a study's strengths and weaknesses.

Dr. Harrington is a global authority on the conduct and interpretation of clinical research. Dr. Lopes joined him 6 years ago, arriving at the Duke Clinical Research Institute to begin his training to become a clinical investigator. They both exemplify the crucial trait of maintaining a presence in clinical care while also developing excellence in the design and conduct of clinical research. Together, they have developed networks of clinicians who conduct research, generate answers, and put them into practice. This cycle of knowledge is the key characteristic of a learning health system in which expertise is gained by participation in the generation of new knowledge through practice. It is particularly noteworthy that this collaboration has evolved into a multinational group focused on developing the next generation of research leaders.

Understanding Clinical Research provides a wonderfully helpful reference for addressing both the operational challenges of clinical trials and the need for an understanding of methods to interpret the results. For those with an interest in pursuing a career in clinical research, this book is an excellent resource to familiarize the reader with the field's history, as well as its contemporary structural and operational components, and major research domains. The chapter authors are all leaders in the field and engaged in cutting-edge clinical research. This experience allows the authors to provide real-life examples to highlight important conceptual issues.

However, this book is not only for researchers but also has equal or more value to the frontline consumers of research, namely students, clinicians, and other healthcare providers. Here the book and its content excel in providing the reader with the tools needed to critically interpret a variety of types of clinical research studies. These include both small and large randomized trials as well as observational research. By reading this book, healthcare providers will be doing themselves and their patients a great service. By actively participating in research and constantly improving practice using the principles contained in this book, readers will be doing an even greater service while also enjoying the benefits of new knowledge and great friendships developed through common research activities.

Robert M. Califf, MD
Donald F. Fortin, MD, Professor of Cardiology and
Professor of Medicine
Duke University School of Medicine
Vice Chancellor for Clinical and Translational Research
Duke University Medical Center
Director, Duke Translational Medicine Institute
Durham, North Carolina

Eric D. Peterson, MD, MPH
Professor of Medicine
Department of Medicine, Division of Cardiology
Duke University School of Medicine
Director, Duke Clinical Research Institute
Durham, North Carolina

Preface

O n behalf of our colleagues and contributors, we are pleased to present this volume. *Understanding Clinical Research* aims to bridge the gap between "cookbooks" and "textbooks" on clinical research—to strike a balance between providing practical information for application as well as broader perspectives that support advancing the field through scholarship.

The first section, Evolution of Clinical Research, places the evolution of the clinical research enterprise in context, from its beginnings in simple everyday observations to its current status as an invaluable global scientific tool. Included in this section are discussions of the rise of information technologies and the academic research organization as integral parts of the research process and the increasing emphasis on and challenges in the ethical conduct of clinical studies.

In the second section, Principles of Clinical Experimentation, readers will find a comprehensive but concise overview of typical phases of clinical research in the development of medical products, from initial exploration of therapeutic effects to monitoring after marketing approval. A standout chapter in this section is devoted to the importance of conducting clinical studies in the pediatric population, which has often been underemphasized in the contemporary literature.

The book's concluding section, Observational Research, reviews the underlying principles, pitfalls, and best practices regarding the conduct of case-control studies, cohort studies, registries, and subgroup analyses within randomized trials. Given the important preponderance of this type of research, especially in an era of "big data" and comparative effectiveness, an informative review of this topic should prove to be of particular value to current and future researchers.

It is our hope that this book can serve as a useful guide for initial reference as well as a springboard for additional investigation. It should also serve as a tribute to the numerous faculty, staff, fellows, and students who have contributed their many talents over the years to make the Duke Clinical Research Institute an outstanding living laboratory for the ongoing conduct and continued study of clinical research and education.

Renato D. Lopes, MD, MHS, PhD
Robert A. Harrington, MD
February 2013

Evolution of Clinical Research

A Brief History of Clinical Trials, Drug Regulations, and the Food and Drug Administration

Nidhi Tripathi, Kate Davis, Catherine Bodine, and Daniel K. Benjamin Jr.

ANCIENT HISTORY

Since early civilizations, people have been concerned about the quality, safety, and integrity of foods and medicines. Curiosity about these matters began thousands of years ago.

In the Bible's Old Testament, the first chapter of the Book of Daniel describes a clinical trial. After conquering Israel, Nebuchadnezzar, the king of Babylon, ordered that several Jewish youths be brought to his palace to serve for 3 years. The children would be fed and taught just like the king's own children. Among the youths was Daniel, who did not wish to defy Jewish law by eating the king's meat or drinking his wine. Daniel asked that the Jewish youth be allowed to eat peas and beans ("pulse") and to drink water instead of wine. Melzar, the eunuch assigned to watch over the youth, was hesitant, fearing Nebuchadnezzr's wrath should Daniel and the other youth become ill. Daniel suggested a 10-day experiment of

3

feeding the Jewish youth pulse and water, while the king's servants continued the rich meats and wine as prescribed by the king.

The result: Daniel 1:15–1:16, King James Version:

*And at the end of ten days their countenances appeared fairer
and fatter in flesh than all the children which did eat the portion
of the king's meat.*

*Thus Melzar took away the portion of their meat, and the wine
that they should drink; and gave them pulse.*

The first known English food law was enacted in 1202, when King John
of England proclaimed the Assize of Bread, a law prohibiting the adulteration of bread with ingredients such as ground peas or beans (1). One of the
earliest food and drug laws in the United States was enacted in 1785, when
the Commonwealth of Massachusetts passed the first general food adulteration law regulating food quality, quantity, and branding.

Since these early times, many events, often accompanied by tragic
outcomes, have raised additional concerns related to food and drug safety.

MODERN HISTORY—THE BEGINNING
OF CLINICAL SCIENCE

As we progressed toward more modern times, clinical trials began using
specific experimental designs and collected information in numbers rather
than in statements such as "looked healthier and better nourished."

One of the earliest examples of an experimental design can be traced to
1767 and William Watson, who was the physician for the Hospital for the
Maintenance and Education of Exposed and Deserted Children in London,
England. At that time, the leading cause of death among children in London
was smallpox, and the governors of the hospital ordered that all children
who were not already immune to smallpox be inoculated. Although inoculation was already an accepted practice, Watson was curious about the benefit
of routinely using mercury as a concomitant treatment with the inoculum.

In October 1767, Watson performed his first experiment, giving 31 children the same inoculum and then dividing them into three similar groups:

- 10 children (5 boys and 5 girls) received a mixture of mercury and
  jalap (a laxative)

- 10 children (5 boys and 5 girls) received an infusion of senna and syrup of roses (a mild laxative)
- 11 boys received no concomitant medicines

Watson understood that he would need to clearly show a lack of efficacy in the use of mercury to convince others to abandon its use. Therefore, he made every effort to create similar groups for comparison. He not only included groups of children of similar ages and both sexes but also demanded that all of the children eat the same diet, wear similar clothes, play in the same fields, and sleep in the same dormitories. In each experiment, the children were inoculated at the same time and place with the same material. Watson understood that "it was proper also to be informed of what nature unassisted, not to say undisturbed, would do for herself" (2). His introduction of an untreated control group, the 11 boys who received no concomitant medicines, was his way of determining the outcome when nature was "unassisted." Watson's method allowed him to compare the results in the three groups (3).

Also during the mid-18th century, James Lind was investigating the cause of and cure for scurvy among seamen. In at least two respects, Lind's *Treatise of the Scurvy* (4) is a good illustration of the basis for mid-18th century judgment and decision making, in that it quotes the contributions of others at length, and its therapeutic recommendations had little impact (5).

When Lind began to read the literature on scurvy, he realized that the only existing descriptions of the disease were written either by seamen who were not doctors or by doctors who had never been to sea. Lind felt that this was one of the reasons why there was so much confusion about the diagnosis, prevention, and cure of the disease.

Although he was a physician, Lind's experiment was not based on pathophysiological theory. He gave no reason for his choice of possible treatments—vinegar, cider, elixir of vitriol, seawater, and lemons and oranges—each of which was given to two seamen. His trial succeeded because one of the treatments contained vitamin C. Lind knew how to perform a comparative experiment and how to control well for time and environment, but he knew perhaps less well which experiment he should do. Had his experiment been based on theory, his work might have been more likely to receive credit with the medical establishment rather than take more than 40 years to be put into practice.

PRECURSORS TO THE FDA IN THE 1800s

The US Food and Drug Administration (FDA), an agency of the Department of Health and Human Services, is charged with the regulation and supervision of most food products, human and animal drugs, biologics, medical devices, cosmetics, and animal feed.

Efforts to protect consumers were first made in the 1800s as early scientific studies continued to develop products for use in humans (Table 1–1). In the 1820s, the first US Pharmacopeia was produced, which set standards for the strength, purity, quality, and consistency of drugs (6). In 1848, Lewis Caleb Beck was appointed to the Patent Office to carry out

TABLE 1–1
Timeline of notable events (6)

Date	Event
1820	Establishment of US Pharmacopeia • First compendium of standard drugs for the United States
1848	Drug Importation Act • In response to the death of American soldiers from adulterated quinine during the Mexican war, requires the US Customs Service to perform inspections to halt entry of adulterated drugs from overseas
1862	Charles M. Wetherill appointed to the Department of Agriculture • Beginning of the Bureau of Chemistry, the predecessor of the Food and Drug Administration
1902	Biologics Control Act • Regulates manufacturers to ensure the purity and safety of serums, vaccines, and other biological products used to prevent or treat diseases in humans
1906	Pure Food and Drugs Act • Prohibits interstate commerce in misbranded and adulterated foods, drinks, and drugs; truth in labeling is required
1912	Sherley Amendment • Prohibits labeling medicines with false therapeutic claims intended to defraud the purchaser; burden of proof lies with the federal government
1937	Elixir of sulfanilamide tragedy • Solution of sulfanilamide in diethylene glycol kills more than 100 people, dramatizing the need to establish drug safety before marketing; impetus to enact the pending food and drug law

TABLE 1–1
Timeline of notable events (6) *(continued)*

Date	Event
1938	Federal Food, Drug, and Cosmetic Act • Requires for the first time that the safety of new drugs be shown before marketing; drugs must be labeled with instructions for safe use, and false claims of efficacy are prohibited
1951	Durham–Humphrey Amendment • Defines the types of drugs that require medical supervision and are for sale by prescription only
1962	Thalidomide causes birth defects • Drug marketed as safe sleeping aid and treatment for morning sickness causes birth defects in thousands of infants born in Western Europe; Dr. Frances Oldham Kelsey prevents the marketing of the drug in the United States Kefauver–Harris Drug Amendment • Requires proof of drug efficacy before marketing, and more stringent requirements for drug safety are adopted; requires some protections of human subjects involved in clinical research, including informed consent Consumer Bill of Rights • President John F. Kennedy proclaims that consumers have the right to safety, the right to be informed, the right to choose, and the right to be heard
1970	FDA requires the first patient package insert • Oral contraceptives must contain information for the patient about specific risks and benefits
1997	Food and Drug Administration Modernization Act (FDAMA) • Offers another 6 months of marketing exclusivity to manufacturers who conduct pediatric drug trials in response to an FDA written request; adds measures to accelerate review of devices, regulate advertising of unapproved uses of approved drugs and devices, and regulate health claims for food
2002	Best Pharmaceuticals for Children Act • Continues 6-month exclusivity provision from FDAMA and establishes a publicly funded method to study off-patent drugs; renewed in 2007
2003	Pediatric Research Equity Act • Gives FDA clear authority to require that manufacturers conduct clinical research into pediatric applications for new drugs and biological products

chemical analyses of agricultural products; many view his appointment as a crucial early step in the development of what is now the FDA. Shortly, thereafter, the Drug Importation Act was passed in response to the deaths of American soldiers from adulterated quinine. This act charged US Customs officers with inspecting and prohibiting the entry of adulterated drugs from overseas.

In 1862, Charles M. Wetherill was appointed chemist for the new Department of Agriculture. This was the beginning of the Bureau of Chemistry, the predecessor to the FDA. Investigations of food adulteration conducted by the Department of Agriculture became fodder for the eventual creation of a food and drug regulatory body. It was not until the United States and Europe suffered a number of tragedies, however, that an official governing board, which eventually became the modern-day FDA, was formed.

DIPHTHERIA ANTITOXIN, TETANUS, AND THE BIOLOGICS CONTROL ACT OF 1902

The late 19th century marked the blooming of international biologics research, leading to the development of new tools for the treatment and prevention of disease (7). In Germany, Robert Koch discovered and isolated the pathogens that cause anthrax, cholera, tuberculosis, and rabies; Louis Pasteur developed a vaccine to protect fowl from cholera in France; and Americans Theobald Smith and Edmund Salmon created heat-killed vaccines to prevent hog cholera.

Soon immunological tools were developed for use in humans. Emil von Behring and Shibasaburo Kitasato, both working in Koch's lab, discovered how to produce and isolate diphtherial and tetanus antitoxin using animal models. The antitoxins were able to both cure and prevent the recurrence of these deadly diseases. Diphtherial antitoxin was tested in human patients in 1891, and the Hoechst pharmaceutical company began commercial production soon thereafter. Serum antitoxin therapy drastically reduced the mortality attributed to diphtheria in Europe, and the Americans took note.

In the United States, diphtherial antitoxin was first produced in the public sector by the Hygienic Laboratory in Washington, DC and the Bacteriological Laboratory of the New York City Health Department. In both instances, horses were immunized to produce large quantities of serum. The private sector quickly developed the expertise necessary to mass-produce serum and vaccines and administer them with sterile syringes. Despite some discussion about the need for regulation and quality control of these biologic products, the private sector operated without oversight.

Tragedy struck in 1901. A 5-year-old girl in St. Louis, Missouri, died from tetanus after being given diphtheria antitoxin serum. Following her death, municipal officials traced the serum to the horse from which it had been produced. Much to their surprise and concern, they learned that the horse had been destroyed after it had contracted tetanus. Rather than discarding the serum isolated from this animal, company officials continued to distribute it to the community; 12 more children died of tetanus in St. Louis. Another 9 children died in New Jersey due to a contaminated smallpox vaccine soon thereafter.

These tragedies prompted Congress to pass the Biologics Control Act of 1902, under which manufacturers were required to be licensed annually to produce and sell vaccines, serums, and antitoxins. Facilities were subject to inspection and could be shut down for noncompliance with regulations. Biologic products were required to be clearly labeled with the product name and expiration date, and a qualified scientist had to oversee production. The 1944 Public Health Service Act extended licensing requirements to biologic products in addition to manufacturers.

PURE FOOD AND DRUGS ACT OF 1906

The adulteration and misbranding of foods and drugs was commonplace at the end of the 19th century (8,9). When Harvey Washington Wiley became the chief chemist in the Division of Chemistry in 1883, he spearheaded the systematic evaluation of chemical preservatives and dyes used in food. A 10-part study entitled *Foods and Food Adulterants*, published from 1887 to 1902, outlined concerns about the impact of chemical preservatives on health. In these studies, preservatives were given to healthy volunteers in increasing amounts, and the responses were observed. The outrage generated by these studies, in addition to revelations about market conditions by journalists such as Samuel Hopkins Adams and novelists such as Upton Sinclair (*The Jungle*), were fuel for the passage of the 1906 Pure Food and Drugs Act.

The Pure Food and Drugs Act, signed into law by President Theodore Roosevelt, prohibited interstate commerce of misbranded or adulterated food, drugs, and drinks at the price of product confiscation or prosecution of the responsible parties. Manufacturers were required to accurately label the contents and dosage of drugs that varied from forms defined in the US Pharmacopoeia and the National Formulary. The act prohibited the adulteration and/or dilution of foods with any substance that could pose a health hazard, and the Bureau of Chemistry was charged with the responsibility of administering these regulations.

The first major test of the legislation came in 1910, when the government seized an ineffective product called Johnson's Mild Combination Treatment for Cancer (10). The Supreme Court ruled in *U.S. v. Johnson* that false claims of effectiveness were not within the purview of the Food and Drugs Act. This loophole was closed in 1912 with the Sherley Amendment, which prohibited labeling with false therapeutic claims to defraud the purchaser. However, the burden of proof that the company intended to defraud the consumer still lay with the government, a task that proved difficult. Of note, the act did not require approval of drugs before marketing, simply truth in labeling.

The Bureau of Chemistry became the Food, Drug, and Insecticide Administration in July 1927, and the FDA in 1931.

ELIXIR OF SULFANILAMIDE 1937–1938

Sulfanilamide was an antibiotic that had successfully and safely treated streptococcal infections for some time (11). Unfortunately, the available pill and powder formulations were not palatable, especially for children. In 1937, the S.E. Massengill Company in Bristol, Tennessee, developed a raspberry-flavored liquid formulation that was distributed across the country. The end product, Elixir of Sulfanilamide, caused the painful deaths of 107 people, mostly children. Although an elixir is an alcohol-based solution, the product sold by Massengill was dissolved in diethylene glycol, a toxic analog of antifreeze. The new formulation had not been tested for toxicity before being widely distributed, so its lethality was unknown.

After learning of these deaths, FDA investigators approached headquarters of the company and discovered that officials had already learned of the toxic effects of their drug. The company had contacted more than 1,000 salesmen, pharmacists, and doctors requesting the return of their product but had conveyed neither a sense of urgency nor information about the toxicity of the solution. The FDA was able to recall the drug from the market, not because of its lethality but because it was incorrectly labeled as an elixir. If not for this technicality, the FDA would have been powerless to act, and many more might have died.

Once again tragedy accelerated legislation. Until this time, there were no requirements to show the safety of a product before it was brought to market. Legislation updating the flawed 1906 Pure Food and Drugs Act, which had been stalled in Congress for 5 years, passed in 1938. Signed into law by President Franklin D. Roosevelt, the Food, Drug, and Cosmetic Act most notably required manufacturers to submit evidence of drug safety to the FDA before the drug could go to market (12). This marked the birth of the new drug application (NDA). Following an NDA submission, the FDA had 2 months to approve, reject, or request additional information before approval was automatically granted. The act further irrefutably prohibited false therapeutic claims, required that drugs be labeled with instructions for safe use, and extended consumer protection to medical devices and cosmetics. The 1951 Durham–Humphrey Amendment required that certain drugs be labeled for sale by prescription only (13).

THALIDOMIDE: MITIGATION OF A EUROPEAN TRAGEDY

Despite the dissemination of the Nuremberg Code outlining ethical practices in human research, in the 1950s and 1960s drug manufacturers still commonly sent doctors unapproved drugs for informal testing on patients without their consent (14). (There was no requirement that the FDA be informed when testing a new drug in humans.) This practice allowed more than 20,000 Americans, including more than 3,000 women of childbearing age and about 200 pregnant women, to be exposed to a drug called thalidomide despite a lack of marketing approval (15).

Thalidomide was manufactured in Germany and marketed as a sleeping aid and antiemetic for morning sickness. It was sold over the counter in Germany in 1957 and throughout Europe by 1960, with the claim that it was completely safe.

So as to introduce thalidomide to the American market, its manufacturer (Chemie Grünenthal) submitted safety studies to the FDA. An FDA medical officer, Frances Oldham Kelsey, was not satisfied by the safety or pharmacokinetic data submitted. Only a few low-quality studies had been performed in the United States, and there were no adequate data on the long-term effects of the drug. Case reports published in the *British Medical Journal* suggesting that peripheral neuropathy developed after chronic thalidomide therapy gave Dr. Kelsey pause. She was particularly concerned with the lack of information about whether the drug could cross the placenta and affect the developing fetus. Approval of the drug for marketing in the United States was stalled because of her misgivings.

Dr. Kelsey's suspicions proved to be correct: more than 10,000 infants in Europe and Africa were born with severe birth defects, most commonly phocomelia—the shortening or absence of limbs. Despite the fact that more than 1,000 physicians were using thalidomide in informal "clinical trials," this tragedy was largely averted in the United States due to Dr. Kelsey's persistence. The narrowly averted thalidomide disaster in the United States led to substantial drug development reform.

The 1962 Kefauver–Harris Amendment led to sweeping reform of the FDA. It required for the first time that manufacturers provide proof of efficacy through adequate and well-controlled trials before marketing a drug. More stringent safety standards were to be enforced, and manufacturers were now required to report adverse events to the FDA. The act also defined ethical standards for the conduct of clinical trials, for example, the requirement for informed consent by the participants. Finally, the FDA now had to specifically approve the marketing application for each drug, and manufacturers were required to disclose the risks and benefits of prescription products to physicians.

CHILDREN: THE NEGLECTED DEMOGRAPHIC 1997

Since the passage of the Kefauver–Harris Amendment, the FDA has been empowered to ensure the safe and efficacious use of drugs in the United States; new drugs must be studied in adequate and well-controlled trials that ultimately form the basis of labels and package inserts detailing safety, efficacy, and directions for use.

The irony of drug development legislation has been that although reforms were spurred largely by tragedies in children, the resulting reform efforts failed to protect children. Despite bearing the brunt of the tragedies that catalyzed the development of regulations, children were excluded from trials that allowed drugs to be brought to market.

By the 1990s, fewer than 15% of drug labels contained information about pediatric dosing, safety, or efficacy. As a result, pediatricians were forced to use these drugs "off-label" and to treat each child as an experiment with a sample size (n) of 1. Neonates and infants were most often neglected in clinical trials because the study of drugs in this population is both technically and ethically challenging. However, the extrapolation of adult or older pediatric safety and dosing information to very young patients is ill advised because of the variable and developing physiology of children. Infants have been victims of unforeseen adverse events, including the development of kernicterus in premature infants treated with prophylactic sulfisoxazole and "gray baby syndrome" resulting from prophylactic chloramphenicol use in the 1950s (16).

The 1997 Food and Drug Administration Modernization Act (FDAMA) provided a financial incentive for pharmaceutical companies to study on-patent drugs in children. It granted an additional 6 months of marketing exclusivity to manufacturers who carried out studies in children in response to an FDA-issued written request. The exclusivity provision was extended under the 2002 Best Pharmaceuticals for Children Act (BPCA) and subsequently renewed in 2007. The BPCA further established a publicly funded mechanism for the study of generic off-patent drugs in children. The Pediatric Research Equity Act (PREA) of 2003 gave the FDA the authority to require drug sponsors to conduct clinical research into pediatric applications of new drugs that may reasonably be used in this population.

FDAMA has successfully stimulated pediatric drug research. Since its enactment in 1997, more than 350 written requests have been issued concerning about 900 studies (17), and there have been 427 labeling changes as of March 2012, mostly attributable to the BPCA or PREA (18). We have learned that simple extrapolation of pharmacokinetic data from adults to children is inadequate, often leading to failed efficacy trials in children not because the drugs are ineffective but because they are not given in appropriate dosages or formulations (19,20).

The increased number of pediatric trials has not resulted in a proportional increase in the number of publications (21,22). The results of only half the studies conducted for additional marketing exclusivity have been published in peer-reviewed journals; those with positive labeling changes are more likely to be published (21). Of particular concern is the small number of safety trials that have been published and the presentation of safety data in a way that is more favorable than the data submitted to the FDA (22). Without widespread publication of trial results, the FDA's review of data produced by the manufacturer in safety, pharmacokinetic, and efficacy trials is the strongest facet of consumer protection and physician guidance.

CONCLUSION

From its humble beginnings as the Department of Agriculture and the 1906 Pure Food and Drugs Act, the modern-day FDA has evolved into an important regulatory body whose jurisdiction encompasses most human and animal food products, drugs, biologics, medical devices, and cosmetics (8). Today, the FDA has a multibillion-dollar budget that it uses to regulate and ensure the safety and efficacy of new products and drugs and to supervise production of $1 trillion worth of products annually.

REFERENCES

1. US Food and Drug Administration. Milestones in U.S. Food and Drug Law History. http://www.fda.gov/AboutFDA/WhatWeDo/History/Milestones/default.htm. Accessed June 27, 2012.
2. Watson W. *An Account of a Series of Experiments, Instituted with a View of Ascertaining the Most Successful Method of Inoculating the Small-Pox.* London: J. Nourse; 1768.
3. Boylston AW. Clinical investigation of smallpox in 1767. *N Engl J Med.* 2002;346(17):1326-1328.
4. Lind J. *A Treatise of the Scurvy.* Edinburgh: Sands, Murray & Cochran; 1753.
5. Tröhler U. Lind and scurvy: 1747 to 1795. *J R Soc Med.* 2005;98(11): 519-522.
6. US Food and Drug Administration. Milestones in U.S. Food and Drug Law History—Significant Dates in U.S. Food and Drug Law History. 2010. http://www.fda.gov/AboutFDA/WhatWeDo/History/Milestones/ucm128305.htm. Accessed April 4, 2012.
7. White Junod S. Selections from FDLI Update Series on FDA History—Biologics Centennial: 100 Years of Biologics Regulation. 2002. http://www.fda.gov/aboutfda/whatwedo/history/productregulation/selectionsfromfdliupdateseriesonfdahistory/ucm091754.htm. Accessed April 4, 2012.
8. Swann JP. FDA's Origin & Functions—FDA's Origin. 2009. http://www.fda.gov/AboutFDA/WhatWeDo/History/Origin/ucm124403.htm. Accessed April 4, 2012.
9. US Food and Drug Administration. FDA's Origin & Functions—FDA History—Part I. 2009. http://www.fda.gov/AboutFDA/WhatWeDo/History/Origin/ucm054819.htm. Accessed April 4, 2012.
10. Meadows M. Promoting Safe and Effective Drugs for 100 Years. http://www.fda.gov/AboutFDA/WhatWeDo/History/ProductRegulation/PromotingSafeandEffective Drugsfor100Years/default.htm. Accessed April 4, 2012.
11. Ballentine C. Sulfanilamide Disaster. 1981. http://www.fda.gov/AboutFDA/WhatWeDo/History/ProductRegulation/ SulfanilamideDisaster/default.htm. Accessed April 4, 2012.

12. US Food and Drug Administration. Summary of NDA Approvals & Receipts, 1938 to the Present. 2011. http://www.fda.gov/AboutFDA/What WeDo/History/ProductRegulation/SummaryofNDAApprovalsReceipt s1938tothepresent/default.htm. Accessed April 4, 2012.
13. US Food and Drug Administration. FDA's Origin & Functions—FDA History—Part III. 2009. http://www.fda.gov/AboutFDA/WhatWeDo/History/ Origin/ucm055118.htm. Accessed April 4, 2012.
14. Liu MB, Davis K. *A Clinical Trials Manual from the Duke Clinical Research Institute: Lessons from a Horse Named Jim*. 2nd ed. Hoboken, NJ: Wiley-Blackwell; 2010.
15. Fintel B, Samaras AT, Carias E. The Thalidomide Tragedy: Lessons for Drug Safety and Regulation & pipe; Science in Society. 2009. http://scienceinsociety.northwestern.edu/content/articles/2009/research-digest/thalidomide/ title-tba. Accessed April 4, 2012.
16. Robertson AF. Reflections on errors in neonatology: II. The "Heroic" years, 1950 to 1970. *J Perinatol*. 2003; 23(2):154-161.
17. US Food and Drug Administration C for DE and R. Development Resources—Breakdown of Requested Studies Report. 2009. http://www.fda. gov/Drugs/DevelopmentApprovalProcess/DevelopmentResources/ ucm050001.htm. Accessed April 4, 2012.
18. US Food and Drug Administration. New Pediatric Labeling Information Database. http://www.accessdata.fda.gov/scripts/sda/sdNavigation.cfm?sd= labelingdatabase. Accessed April 4, 2012.
19. Dunne J, et al. Extrapolation of adult data and other data in pediatric drug-development programs. *Pediatrics*. 2011; 128(5):e1242-e1249.
20. Benjamin DK Jr, et al. Pediatric antihypertensive trial failures: analysis of end points and dose range. *Hypertension*. 2008;51(4):834-840.
21. Benjamin DK Jr, et al. Peer-reviewed publication of clinical trials completed for pediatric exclusivity. *JAMA*. 2006;296(10):1266-1273.
22. Benjamin DK Jr, et al. Safety and transparency of pediatric drug trials. *Arch Pediatr Adolesc Med*. 2009;163(12): 1080-1086.

CHAPTER TWO

Information Technology, Access, ClinicalTrials .gov

Anjan K. Chakrabarti and C. Michael Gibson

INFORMATION TECHNOLOGY AND CLINICAL RESEARCH

In the late 20th and early 21st centuries, concern grew among scientists, clinicians, and public policymakers regarding the direction of clinical research. Over the previous five decades, the scientific community had benefited from significant progress in the realm of basic science research, backed by the public's long-term investment in it. The concern over clinical research stemmed from the idea that scientific discoveries of these past generations were not being appropriately translated. This was addressed with numerous targeted initiatives, including the Clinical Research Roundtable at the Institute of Medicine in June 2000. This initiative identified four major challenges to the progress of clinical research: (1) enhancing public participation in clinical research, (2) funding, (3) an adequately trained workforce, and (4) developing information systems (1). The last challenge mentioned, and the focus of this section, highlights the idea that the use of information technology (IT) and standards not only improves healthcare delivery, accuracy, and patient safety (2) but also advances clinical research.

Information technology has now been integrated into every phase of clinical research. Physician–investigators use IT to assist in designing of

17

hypotheses and protocols, identifying and recruiting research subjects, implementing data collection instruments, training research staff, ensuring regulatory compliance, and generating timely reports (1,3). IT applications have been tailored to both research and clinical systems; both have influenced the world of clinical research with considerable overlap (Figure 2–1) (4).

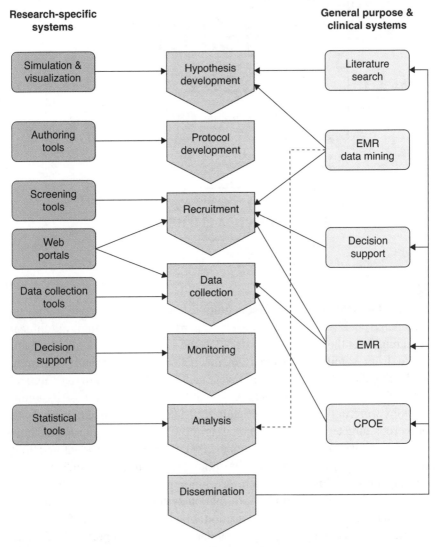

FIGURE 2–1. Information technology systems supporting the translational research enterprise. CPOE, computerized physician order entry; EMR, electronic medical record. Reproduced, with permission, from Payne PRO, Johnson SB, Starren JB, Tilson HH, Dowdy D. Breaking the translational barriers: The value of integrating biomedical informatics and translational research. *J Investig Med*. 2005;53(4):192-200.

TABLE 2–1

**Research-specific information technology systems
and their utility in clinical research**

IT system	Application in clinical research
Simulation and visualization tools	Streamline the preclinical research process (e.g., disease models) and assist in the analysis of complex datasets
Protocol authorizing tools	Allow collaborating authors to work on complex protocols regardless of geographic location
Research-specific Web portals	Allow researchers a single point of access for research information and collaboration
Electronic data collection/capture tools	Organize research-specific data in a structured form, reduce redundancies and errors occurring with paper-based data collection

Clinical IT systems have made an enormous impact on clinical research and study design (5). Specifically, hypothesis development and study preparation have been enhanced by the ability to perform literature searches using tools such as PubMed (6). Cohort identification and study recruitment have been enhanced by data-mining tools, and decision support systems, including clinical trial alert systems, have helped identify study candidates (7,8). The electronic medical record has streamlined clinical data collection from research participants, reduced redundant data entry, and helped identify patients who qualify for clinical investigations; in addition, computerized physician order entry has allowed accurate tracking of therapies prescribed and delivered to study patients (9,10).

In addition to clinical IT systems, several research-specific IT systems have been developed that have led to increases in data and research quality. These are now being implemented in clinical research studies at growing rates (6,11). Table 2–1 outlines some of the research-specific IT systems and their utility in clinical research (12–16).

IT systems and their application in clinical research have continued to evolve; Embi and colleagues proposed in 2009 that a new domain had emerged in medical informatics, referred to as clinical research informatics (17). They defined this new domain as:

... the subdomain of biomedical informatics concerned with the development, application, and evaluation of theories, methods, and systems to optimize the design and conduct of clinical

research and the analysis, interpretation, and dissemination of the information generated.

Naturally, with the evolution of clinical research informatics and the development of large, integrated datasets, it became easier to pursue the idea of clinical trial registries, in which data from human trials could be available for mass consumption. Previously, the idea of clinical trial registries was met with many barriers and challenges, including the extensive resources needed to create and maintain the registries, the need to agree on standard data elements, the ability to manage data from multiple sources, the ability to regularly update and keep data accurate and complete, and proprietary/technical concerns (18). These challenges were addressed by the ever-changing idea of clinical research informatics, which led to next great debate in clinical research: To register or not to register?

ACCESS TO CLINICAL RESEARCH AND CLINICALTRIALS.GOV

The emergence of IT led to the rapid progression of clinical research and generation of massive amounts of data from human research subjects. While this was happening, concern developed in the medical and scientific communities that although clinical trials now had the potential to improve medical practice, significant access barriers persisted that created a gap between research and practice. This was eloquently suggested by Haynes and colleagues in 1998, who pointed to the volume and complexity of research being conducted and poor access to it as a significant barrier to practicing evidence-based medicine (19). The idea of registering clinical trials was picking up steam and supported by investigators such as Smith and colleagues, who in 1997 actually called for an "amnesty" for unpublished trials. Not surprisingly, they received a disappointing response (20).

Individual registries of small data did exist before 1998. A survey conducted by Easterbrook and colleagues in 1989 revealed 24 registries, including the internal registry of thrombosis and hemostasis trials and the Oxford Perinatal Trial Registry (21); there were also government-supported systems, including the AIDS Clinical Trials Information Service (ACTIS) and CancerNet (18). Over the next 10 years, more fragmented registries would develop, but they would continue to be limited by variance in recorded details and nonadherence to a standard of accuracy and comprehensiveness.

Several patient advocacy groups began to argue that clinical trials and their results should be made available to the public. This movement led to passage of the 1997 Food and Drug Administration Modernization Act (FDAMA), in which Section 113 required creation of a database of information about clinical trials. Specifically, it called for:

A registry of clinical trials (whether federally or privately funded) of experimental treatments for serious or life-threatening diseases and conditions . . . which provides a description of the purpose of each experimental drug, either with the consent of the protocol sponsor, or when a trial to test effectiveness begins. Information provided shall consist of eligibility criteria for participation in the clinical trials, a description of the location of trial sites, and a point of contact for those wanting to enroll in the trial, and shall be in a form that can be readily understood by members of the public. (22)

Thus, ClinicalTrials.gov was born. It was established in 2000 by the National Library of Medicine on behalf of the National Institutes of Health (NIH) (23). Initially, sponsors were required to register only clinical trials assessing drugs for treatment of serious or life-threatening illnesses; even with this limited scope, compliance was found to be poor (24). It was not until 2004 that two events precipitated increased compliance in reporting and registration.

The first was in June, when New York State sued GlaxoSmithKline for failing to publish the negative results of a trial of paroxetine in pediatric patients. The second, and perhaps most significant to date, was the policy set forth by the International Committee of Medical Journal Editors (25). They announced that effective in 2005 (implemented on September 13, 2005), that reports of clinical trials would be accepted for publication only if the trial had been properly registered. The results of this decision were staggering: an observational study by Zarin and colleagues showed that registrations increased by 73% between May and October 2005, from 13,153 to 22,714 trials (Figure 2–2) (26). This increase in registrations was associated with a 195% increase in the number of data providers from around the world (26).

Even with the large increase in registered trials after the 2005 policy decision, there remained a large degree of publication bias, or the selective publication of positive research studies, as well as outcome reporting bias, which includes selective reporting of outcomes within a publication. This

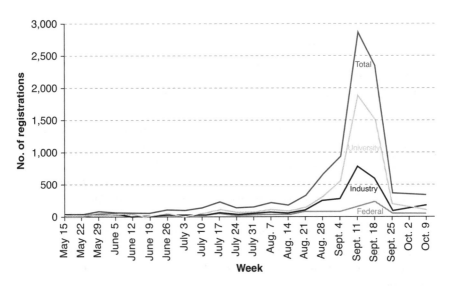

FIGURE 2–2. New trials registered at ClinicalTrials.gov between May and October 2005. Reproduced, with permission, from Zarin DA, Tse T, Ide NC. Trial Registration at ClinicalTrials.gov between May and October 2005. *N Engl J Med.* 2005; 353(26):2779-2787.

prompted passage of the FDA Amendments Act of 2007 (FDAAA), which expanded the scope of clinical trial registration and added new requirements for reporting results to ClinicalTrials.gov.

Specifically, this new law required study sponsors or principal investigators to report summary results for interventional studies of "drugs, biologic products, and devices within 1 year of completing data collection for the prespecified primary outcome, regardless of sponsor or funding source" (24,27). This spawned creation of the ClinicalTrials.gov Results Database in September 2008, which allowed data providers to report summary results of clinical trials and observational studies in a tabular format. This latest innovation created a public record of basic study results, thus promoting the ethical responsibility of researchers, mitigating the above-mentioned selection and publication biases, and facilitating systematic reviews.

As of the writing of this chapter, ClinicalTrials.gov has registered 129,733 trials with locations in 174 countries (28). This highlights the strides that have been made in public access to clinical research and the profound impact that IT development has had in moving clinical research forward. Although the challenges identified by the Clinical Research

Roundtable at the Institute of Medicine in June 2000 may still exist, significant progress has been made in the last two decades.

FUTURE DIRECTIONS

The climate in which clinical research is being conducted continues to change and evolve. Now, in 2012, patient enrollment and recruitment occur globally, and many large trials are being sponsored by industry, amplifying a potential "credibility gap" (29). In addition, sources of medical data are becoming more heterogeneous, particularly in the United States, where a central electronic medical record has not been adopted by most primary care providers and hospitals (30). Moving forward, sophisticated IT systems will be needed to ensure the quality of data used in clinical research, the transparency with which those data are collected and analyzed, and the efficiency with which they can be collected. This may indeed be a challenge, given that the adoption of IT applications for clinical research has been variable, particularly among academic medical centers in the United States (31). Perhaps the only way to ensure that IT and clinical research evolve together is with significant investments in health informatics and IT infrastructure.

KEY POINTS

- The Clinical Research Roundtable at the Institute of Medicine in June 2000 highlighted the importance of the development of IT systems to the progress of clinical research.
- Both clinical IT and research-specific IT systems affect each phase of the modern clinical research study.
- The FDA Modernization Act in 1997, Section 113, required the creation of a database of information about clinical trials.
- In 2000, the National Library of Medicine established ClinicalTrials.gov on behalf of the NIH.
- Registration of new trials increased significantly after the September 2005 ICMJE requirement for registration before publication.
- Creation of the ClinicalTrials.gov Results Database in September 2008 helped mitigate both publication and selection biases.

REFERENCES

1. Sung NS, et al. Central challenges facing the national clinical research enterprise. *JAMA*. 2003;289(10):1278-1287.
2. McDonald CJ, Schadow G, Suico J, Overhage JM. Data standards in health care. *Ann Emerg Med*. 2001;38(3):303-311.
3. Grimes DA, Schulz KF. An overview of clinical research: the lay of the land. *Lancet*. 2002;359(9300):57-61.
4. Payne PRO, Johnson SB, Starren JB, Tilson HH, Dowdy D. Breaking the translational barriers: the value of integrating biomedical informatics and translational research. *J Investig Med*. 2005;53(4):192-200.
5. Embi PJ, Kaufman SE, Payne PRO. Biomedical informatics and outcomes research: enabling knowledge-driven health care. *Circulation*. 2009;120(23): 2393-2399.
6. Briggs B. Clinical trials getting a hand. *Health Data Manag*. 2002;10(2): 56-60, 62.
7. Marks L, Power E. Using technology to address recruitment issues in the clinical trial process. *Trends Biotechnol*. 2002;20(3):105-109.
8. Embi PJ, et al. Effect of a clinical trial alert system on physician participation in trial recruitment. *Arch Intern Med*. 2005;165(19):2272-2277.
9. Bates DW, Ebell M, Gotlieb E, Zapp J, Mullins HC. A proposal for electronic medical records in U.S. primary care. *J Am Med Inform Assoc*. 2003; 10(1):1-10.
10. Teich JM, et al. Effects of computerized physician order entry on prescribing practices. *Arch Intern Med*. 2000;160(18):2741-2747.
11. Marks RG, Conlon M, Ruberg SJ. Paradigm shifts in clinical trials enabled by information technology. *Stat Med*. 2001;20(17-18):2683-2696.
12. Fazi P, Grifoni P, Luzi D, Ricci FL, Vignetti M. Is workflow technology suitable to represent and manage clinical trials? *Stud Health Technol Inform*. 2000;77:302-306.
13. Holford NH, Kimko HC, Monteleone JP, Peck CC. Simulation of clinical trials. *Annu Rev Pharmacol Toxicol*. 2000; 40:209-234.
14. Rubin DL, Gennari J, Musen MA. Knowledge representation and tool support for critiquing clinical trial protocols. *Proc AMIA Symp*. 2000:724-728.
15. Tai BC, Seldrup J. A review of software for data management, design and analysis of clinical trials. *Ann Acad Med Singapore*. 2000;29(5):576-581.
16. Westgren M, Kublickas M. To use Internet in collaborative studies and registers. *Acta Obstet Gynecol Scand*. 2000;79(5):329-330.
17. Embi PJ, Payne PRO. Clinical research informatics: challenges, opportunities and definition for an emerging domain. *J Am Med Inform Assoc*. 2009; 16(3):316-327.

18. McCray AT. Better access to information about clinical trials. *Ann Intern Med.* 2000;133(8):609-614.
19. Haynes B, Haines A. Barriers and bridges to evidence based clinical practice. *BMJ.* 1998;317(7153):273-276.
20. Roberts I, Hoey J. An amnesty for unpublished trials. *CMAJ.* 1997;157(11): 1548.
21. Easterbrook PJ. Directory of registries of clinical trials. *Stat Med.* 1992; 11(3):363-423.
22. US Food and Drug Administration. FDA Plan for Statutory Compliance. 1998. http://www.fda.gov/Regulatory Information/Legislation/Federal FoodDrugand Cosmeti cActFDCAct/SignificantAmendmentstotheFDCAct/ FDAMA/FDAPlanforStatutoryCompliance/default.htm. Accessed April 4, 2012.
23. McCray AT, Ide NC. Design and implementation of a national clinical trials registry. *J Am Med Inform Assoc.* 2000;7(3):313-323.
24. Miller JD. Registering clinical trial results: the next step. *JAMA.* 2010; 303(8):773-774.
25. International Committee of Medical Journal Editors. Uniform Requirements for Manuscripts Submitted to Biomedical Journals. 2010. http://www.icmje. org/urm_full.pdf. Accessed October 31, 2011.
26. Zarin DA, Tse T, Ide NC. Trial Registration at ClinicalTrials.gov between May and October 2005. *N Engl J Med.* 2005;353(26):2779-2787.
27. Tse T, Williams RJ, Zarin DA. Reporting "basic results" in ClinicalTrials. gov. *Chest.* 2009;136(1):295-303.
28. National Institutes of Health. Home-ClinicalTrials.gov. http://clinicaltrials. gov/. Accessed April 4, 2012.
29. Pyke S, et al. The potential for bias in reporting of industry-sponsored clinical trials. *Pharm Stat.* 2011;10(1):74-79.
30. Jha AK, Doolan D, Grandt D, Scott T, Bates DW. The use of health information technology in seven nations. *Int J Med Inform.* 2008;77(12):848-854.
31. Murphy SN, et al. Current state of information technologies for the clinical research enterprise across academic medical centers. *Clin Transl Sci.* 2012; 5(3):281-284.

CHAPTER THREE

The Role of Academic Research Organizations in Clinical Research

Craig J. Reist, Tyrus L. Rorick, Lisa G. Berdan, and Renato D. Lopes

INTRODUCTION

The label *academic research organization* (ARO), used broadly within the clinical and drug development industries, primarily refers to an academic and/or nonprofit institution that performs one or more functions in the conduct of clinical trials. The services that an ARO provides can range from academic leadership to full-service clinical trial management capabilities, including site monitoring, data management, statistical analysis, safety monitoring, and clinical events classification, in addition to clinical expertise.

The concept of an ARO dates back several decades, when researchers recognized the need for large global clinical trials to answer important medical questions. Clinical scientists from several of the world's leading academic institutions formed teams of like-minded investigators with the goal of developing and conducting global clinical studies to improve patient care. AROs are focused on developing and sharing knowledge with the end goal of improving patient care. They accomplish this goal not only by leading and conducting multinational clinical trials but also by ensuring that the results from these trials are published and presented. These groups also focus on managing major national patient registries designed to collect data and determine best practices, which can then be incorporated into clinical practice guidelines. Education and development of clinical investigators is also a focus, with many of the leading AROs having fellowship programs whose influence extends around the globe.

THE EARLY YEARS

The concept of the ARO dates back to the late 1980s, when several groups of physician investigators first came together to address unmet clinical needs by organizing and centralizing the operational efforts associated with conducting large multicenter clinical trials, so-called "megatrials." The first such group, located at the University of Oxford in the United Kingdom, developed in 1975 from a single research team. It began enrollment of the then-largest trial in history—6,027 patients with suspected acute myocardial infarction (MI)—in mid-1981, completed enrollment at the 245 participating coronary care units in 1985, and published the results the next year (1). Similarly, the Gruppo Italiano per lo Studio della Sopravvivenza nell'Infarto Miocardico (GISSI), formed from a collaboration between the Mario Negri Institute and the Associazione Nazionale dei Medici Cardiologi Ospedalieri, began enrolling 11,806 patients with acute MI in 176 Italian intensive care units in 1984. It published the study results 2 years later (2). Both groups have since continued to perform large, important multicenter trials.

Two groups in particular have paved the way for what we now know as AROs. The Thrombolysis In Myocardial Infarction (TIMI) study group, based in Boston, Massachusetts, and affiliated with Brigham and Women's Hospital and Harvard Medical School, was among the first groups to take on the challenges associated with organizing and implementing global clinical trials (3). The TIMI series of trials began in 1984, initially sponsored by the National Heart, Lung, and Blood Institute (NHLBI). At first, the trials studied thrombolytic and antithrombotic therapies in patients with acute MI and unstable angina, but they now cover many aspects of cardiovascular disease.

Around the same time, other groups of academic investigators were beginning to organize their efforts to address important clinical questions, and thought leaders from around the world formed an alliance to facilitate the conduct of pivotal cardiovascular clinical trials. The VIrtual Coordinating Centre for Global CollabOrative CardiovascUlar Research (VIGOUR) is a working group of global thought leaders in cardiovascular clinical medicine who have achieved academic and industry recognition for performing large multinational clinical trials. The alliance developed from a group of academic investigators participating in the international Global Utilization of Streptokinase and TPA (alteplase) for Occluded Coronary Arteries (GUSTO-1) trial, which began enrollment in 1990 (4). VIGOUR members have since conducted many large international trials, all according to the group's philosophical perspectives on clinical trial design and methods (5). The VIGOUR organization is committed to improving the practice of cardiovascular medicine and patient outcomes (6).

During the 1990s and into the new millennium, many more now-prominent AROs began to formalize their efforts to lead the development of new therapeutics and shape the future of clinical practice across the globe. Table 3–1 lists some of the major AROs currently leading clinical trials (7), and Figure 3–1 displays their global distribution.

ARO VALUES AND PRINCIPLES

Although each ARO has unique characteristics, they share some common values and principles. In general, AROs are nonprofit organizations dedicated to quality research based on high standards and scientific integrity. The operational services that these groups perform comply with Good Clinical Practice guidelines and adhere to national and international regulations. The groups strive to ensure that the questions being asked are important clinical questions that will lead to new therapeutics and improved patient care, regardless of the outcome of the trial. Critical to the academic mission of these organizations is the dissemination of new knowledge to the clinical community and patient population being studied (8). Revenue margins are used to fund unfunded or underfunded

TABLE 3–1
Major academic research organizations

Organization	Location
Brazilian Clinical Research Institute (BCRI)	São Paulo, Brazil
Canadian VIGOUR Centre (CVC)	Edmonton, Alberta, Canada
Cleveland Clinic Cardiovascular Coordinating Center (C5) Research	Cleveland, Ohio, USA
Colorado Prevention Center (CPC)	Denver, Colorado, USA
Duke Clinical Research Institute (DCRI)	Durham, North Carolina, USA
Flinders Coordinating Centre	Adelaide, South Australia, Australia
George Institute	Sydney, New South Wales, Australia
Green Lane Coordinating Centre	Auckland, New Zealand
Leuven Coordinating Centre	Leuven, Belgium
McMaster University	Hamilton, Ontario, Canada
Medanta	New Delhi, India
Montreal Heart Institute	Montreal, Québec, Canada
National Health and Medical Research Council	Sydney, New South Wales, Australia
Nottingham Clinical Research Limited	Nottingham, United Kingdom
TIMI Study Group (TIMI)	Boston, Massachusetts, USA
University of Oxford Clinical Trial Service Unit	Oxford, United Kingdom
Uppsala Clinical Research Center (UCR)	Uppsala, Sweden

Source: Adapted, with permission, from Harrington RA, Califf RM, Hodgson PK, Peterson ED, Roe MT, Mark DB. Careers for clinician investigators. *Circulation*. 2009;119(22):2945-2950.

trials that often address key clinical questions unrelated to commercial development of a drug or device. The results obtained from ARO trials undergo rigorous analyses, and the knowledge gained is incorporated into clinical practice guidelines and supports evidence-based medicine around the globe.

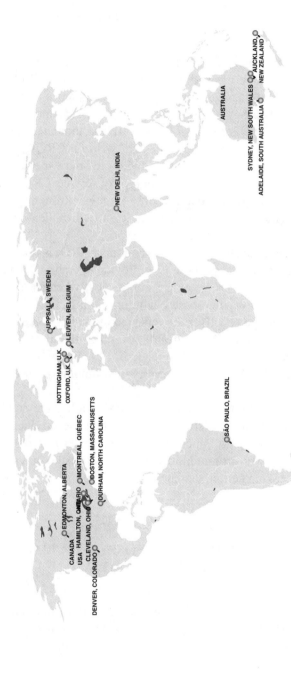

FIGURE 3–1. Global distribution of the academic research organizations listed in Table 3–1.

COMPARING AND CONTRASTING
CROs AND AROs

Much of the research being conducted around the world is currently being managed by contract or clinical research organizations (CROs). CROs typically provide trial management services for companies in the pharmaceutical and biotechnology industries. These services can include preclinical research, clinical research, clinical trials management and/or monitoring, data management, and medical writing. CROs range from large (several thousand employees worldwide) to small specialty groups focused on a particular therapeutic area or type of service. CROs market to their clients that they can move a new drug or device from conception to regulatory and marketing approval more efficiently than the company can using its own staff for these services.

A primary difference between CROs and most AROs is that CROs are for-profit companies whose purpose is to provide operational services for their clients, typically pharmaceutical companies, whereas the primary focus of an ARO is knowledge-based, with improving clinical care as the goal. These different perspectives are reflected in the mission and purpose statements available on the Web sites of several of the major CROs and AROs (see Table 3–2). Another difference is a greater emphasis on collaboration among AROs, which is less typical among often-competing CROs (9).

AROs not only believe that they are responsible for the conduct and quality of each trial but also strive to ensure that the products of their research activities result in enhanced knowledge and improved patient care. This is done by ensuring clinical input in the design and operations of trials and by making certain that the results are published for the healthcare community at large.

ARO COMMITMENT TO EDUCATION
AND TRAINING

A primary goal of any academic organization is education and training. AROs pride themselves on being institutions where future investigators can come to learn clinical research methods, leading to responsible research.

The Duke Clinical Research Institute
as a Model ARO

The inception of the Duke Clinical Research Institute (DCRI) dates from 1969 with the formation of the Duke Databank for Cardiovascular Disease, a research group within Duke University Medical Center. The Databank was the result of an idea of then-Chairman of Medicine, Eugene A. Stead, Jr., MD, who envisioned it as a "computerized textbook of medicine," using information gathered by one physician today to help other physicians care for similar patients tomorrow.

Since 1969, data from all patients undergoing invasive cardiac procedures at Duke have been entered into the Databank, which has since been expanded to include noninvasive diagnostic procedures. Patients with a diagnosis of coronary artery disease are followed annually throughout their lives. Follow-up of the >130,000 patients in the Databank continues today and is more than 99% complete. The continuous maintenance of the Databank for nearly 35 years has given DCRI faculty and staff extensive experience with a long-term follow-up system, including ascertainment of hospital records. The Databank is the world's oldest and largest cardiovascular database.

In the mid-1980s, the research team began to coordinate multicenter clinical trials. The group used its clinical expertise to help design well-crafted protocols and its biostatistics expertise to determine appropriate trial designs and sample sizes to answer the questions addressed in the protocols. The group's landmark trial began in 1990: GUSTO-1, a 4-arm study of thrombolytic therapies that enrolled 41,021 patients with acute MI in 1081 hospitals in 15 countries (4). As noted above, GUSTO-1 gave rise not only to the VIGOUR collaboration but also to a variety of multinational randomized trials in which global academic leaders played increasingly pivotal roles. Today these academic partners often serve as principal investigators, while the DCRI provides operational expertise in jointly designed clinical research projects.

In addition to designing, managing, and analyzing clinical trials, the DCRI also has extensive capabilities in outcomes research and has incorporated cost-effectiveness and quality-of-life assessments into many megatrials. The DCRI has also become increasingly involved in managing data warehouses and conducting registries and clinical trials in collaboration with professional medical societies and the National Institutes of Health.

To date, the DCRI has completed more than 760 Phase I–IV clinical trials, registries, and economics/outcomes studies comprising more than 1 million subjects from 65 countries (10). The organization employs 1100

TABLE 3–2

Mission/purpose statements of major academic/contract research organizations

Academic research organizations		Contract research organizations	
Organization	Mission/purpose statement	Organization	Mission/purpose statement
Brazilian Clinical Research Institute (BCRI)	To develop and share knowledge that improves the care, health, and quality of life of patients in Brazil and Latin America through innovative clinical research while contributing meaningfully to the improvement of patient care around the world.	Covance Inc.	Our mission is to help our clients bring the miracles of medicine to market sooner.
Cleveland Clinic Coordinating Center for Clinical Research (C5Research)	The C5Research mission is to design and conduct innovative clinical research that enhances scientific knowledge about the treatment of diseases and improves medical care of patients.	ICON plc	Our goal is to provide exceptional services to complete our clients' clinical trials.
Canadian VIrtual coordinating center for Global cOllaborative cardiovascUlar Research (VIGOUR) Centre (CVC)	The mission of the Canadian VIGOUR Centre is to be recognized locally, nationally, and internationally, as a leader in cardiovascular research; to be a partner with the University of Alberta to enhance the University's reputation as one of the world's finest research, teaching, and community service institutions; and to be recognized within the University of Alberta as a centre of innovation that is dedicated to the achievement of this mission.	Parexel International Corp.	Parexel's mission is to combine the strength of our expertise, experience and innovation to advance the worldwide success of the bio/pharmaceutical and medical device industries in preventing and curing disease.

Colorado Prevention Center (CPC)	We are dedicated to improving health through clinical research and integrating evidence into community prevention programs.
Duke Clinical Research Institute (DCRI)	Our mission is to develop and share knowledge that improves the care of patients around the world through innovative clinical research.
Greenlane Coordinating Centre	Our mission is to improve the health and quality of life of people throughout the world through innovative clinical research.
Thrombolysis In Myocardial Infarction (TIMI) Study Group	Since its inception in 1984, the principal goal of the TIMI Study Group has been to conduct high-quality clinical trials that enhance the care of patients with coronary artery disease.
Uppsala Clinical Research Center (UCR)	The overarching objective of UCR is to develop and enhance health and medical care by providing service in clinical research, clinical trials, quality registries, and quality development.
Pharmaceutical Product Development, LLC (PPD)	Our mission is to help our clients and partners in maximizing returns on their R&D investment.
Quintiles Transnational Corp.	Quintiles helps to improve healthcare worldwide by providing a broad range of professional services, information and partnering solutions to the pharmaceutical, biotechnology and healthcare industries.

faculty and staff and occupies almost 150,000 square feet of space within and around the Duke University Medical Center campus. As an Institute of the Medical Center, it is a fully integrated component of the university, governed by the Duke University Health System Board of Trustees, which in turn reports to the University Board of Trustees.

CONCLUSION

Clearly, more can be done as we move forward, including closer networking of academic groups, ensuring value to both commercial and academic partners, and ensuring that academic groups commit to and deliver results that rival any large CRO.

The history of the DCRI shows the ability of an ARO to incorporate both new initiatives and new capabilities to meet the needs of an evolving clinical research enterprise. Whether the aim is to know the risks and benefits of a new therapy, to measure the cost-effectiveness of an existing technique, or to integrate the most appropriate patient care into the practice of every physician, AROs such as the DCRI constantly reassess their abilities to respond to the evolving needs of the healthcare system.

REFERENCES

1. First International Study of Infarct Survival Collaborative Group. Randomised trial of intravenous atenolol among 16027 cases of suspected acute myocardial infarction: ISIS-1. *Lancet.* 1986;2(8498):57-66.
2. Gruppo Italiano per lo Studio della Streptochinasi nell'Infarto Miocardico (GISSI). Effectiveness of intravenous thrombolytic treatment in acute myocardial infarction. *Lancet.* 1986;1(8478):397-402.
3. TIMI Study Group. About TIMI Study Group. http://www.timi.org/?page_id=97. Accessed April 5, 2012.
4. The GUSTO Investigators. An international randomized trial comparing four thrombolytic strategies for acute myocardial infarction. *N Engl J Med.* 1993;329(10):673-682.
5. Topol EJ, et al. Perspectives on large-scale cardiovascular clinical trials for the new millennium. The Virtual Coordinating Center for Global Collaborative Cardiovascular Research (VIGOUR) Group. *Circulation.* 1997;95(4):1072-1082.
6. Armstrong PW, Kaul P. Charting the course of clinical research: from an inspired past to a promising future. *Am Heart J.* 2004;148(2):190-192.

7. Harrington RA, et al. Careers for clinician investigators. *Circulation*. 2009; 119(22):2945-2950.

8. Carayol N, Matt M. Does research organization influence academic production? Laboratory level evidence from a large European university. *Res Policy*. 2004;33(8):1081-1102.

9. Shuchman M. Commercializing clinical trials–risks and benefits of the CRO boom. *N Engl J Med*. 2007;357(14):1365-1368.

10. Duke Clinical Research Institute. DCRI Annual Report, 2011. https://dcri.org/about-us/resolveuid/16abf2791474beb759324d47db642ee1. Accessed April 5, 2012.

CHAPTER FOUR

Ethics of Clinical Research: An Overview and Emerging Issues

Yee Weng Wong and Kevin A. Schulman

INTRODUCTION

Clinical research has been pivotal in improving human health over the last century. Understanding of human biology and therapeutic innovation are direct results of sound clinical research involving human volunteers. Responsible and careful planning and implementation of research protocols, guided by ethical values and principles, safeguard the very people that the research is intended to benefit. In this chapter, we provide a brief overview of the ethical principles underlying clinical research and the historical context that shapes current standards. We then address practical applications of these principles and explore emerging issues.

What Is Clinical Research?

Human subjects protection is the centerpiece of clinical research ethics. In most countries, it is regulated by sets of laws and regulations that are shaped by ethical principles, but these form the bare minimal requirements of clinical research ethics. To understand the application of ethical values to clinical research, it is useful to consider the definition and scope of clinical research.

Research is a "systematic investigation, including research development, testing and evaluation, designed to develop or contribute to generalizable knowledge" (1). Clinical research is research that directly involves a person or group of people or material of human origin (such as tissues, specimens, or cognition) for which a researcher either interacts directly with human subjects or collects identifiable private information. Under US regulations, in vitro studies using human tissue not linked to a living person are excluded from the definition (2).

Clinical research can be further subdivided into patient-oriented research, epidemiological and behavioral studies, and outcomes and health services research. Patient-oriented research includes research on disease, therapeutic interventions, clinical trials, and development of biotechnologies. From a bioethics perspective, patient-oriented clinical research is the most vulnerable form of clinical research, because the use of human subjects is the basis of the experimental exercise. Participants in clinical research accept risks and inconvenience, often without obtaining direct benefit from their participation, mainly to advance science and benefit others. Therefore, for persons to be willing to participate and for funding to be provided for such research, the design, implementation, and dissemination of findings must be conducted according to the highest ethical standards.

Current understanding of clinical research ethics is guided by several codes of conduct, often the legacies of tragedies in unethical human subjects research (see Chapter 1). These codes of conduct include the Nuremberg Code (3), the Declaration of Helsinki (4), the Belmont Report (5), and the International Conference on Harmonisation Guidances on Good Clinical Practices (ICH-GCP) (6). In the United States, titles 21 and 45 of the Code of Federal Regulations (CFR) (1) provide guidance for human subjects research. To gain a better understanding of these principles, it is important to consider their historical context.

Beginnings of Clinical Research Ethics

As discussed in Chapter 1, one of the earliest clinical research projects was the study of scurvy attributed to James Lind, a British Royal Navy surgeon in the mid-1700s (7). In addition to Lind's contribution to medical science of controlled experimentation methods, his practice of experimental observation was novel at the time. The notion of performing experiments directly on human subjects to determine the cause of diseases and superiority of treatment options was certainly not the norm and, to most people at the time, simply immoral.

This attitude persisted for more than a century and led to scrutiny of early human experiments in microbiology and immunology by Edward Jenner, Louis Pasteur, and Walter Reed. In Reed's classic experiments on yellow fever transmission, he and his colleague, Jesse William Lazear, intentionally inoculated healthy subjects who had volunteered. All of the subjects were willful participants who were informed of the risks and purpose of the experiments, set out in written documents signed by each volunteer. This early example of written informed consent was viewed by some of his contemporaries as adequate to justify its morality (8,9). However, the modern concept of informed consent in clinical research would be cemented only after tragedies occurred decades later. The key incidents shaping our modern conception of research bioethics include the Tuskegee syphilis study, the Nuremberg trials, and the Willowbrook hepatitis study.

Tuskegee Study

The Tuskegee syphilis study, conducted by the US Public Health Service in Macon County, Alabama, has become a classic case study for bioethics in clinical research. The study started in 1932 with a goal of studying the natural history of untreated syphilis. African American men were the research subjects. This observational study continued until 1972 without offering widely available penicillin as treatment to the participants. The study ended only after a news report in the *Washington Star* drew public attention. Although public debate about the study included allegations of racism as a motivation, several bioethical violations were highlighted in this case. First, the men in the study were recruited from a socially disadvantaged rural community. They were misled or coerced into the study under the impression that the study visits and procedures were part of free treatments and health checks that would otherwise not be available to them. Furthermore, subjects were not given adequate information about the potential hazards and long-term consequences of untreated syphilis to provide informed consent for participation. Most important, the researchers insisted on continuing the trial and withholding effective treatment for syphilis, even after the efficacy of treatment and long-term complications of the condition were known (10,11).

Nuremberg Trial

At the conclusion of World War II, the atrocities committed against concentration camp inmates by Nazi doctors in the form of inhumane experiments were brought to light during the 1947 Nuremberg Military Tribunal. Twenty-three doctors and scientists were brought to trial, and 15 were convicted (12,13). The tribunal's final judgment included a 10-point statement, later known as the Nuremberg Code, that delineated permissible medical experimentation on human subjects. The code can be summarized as follows, with voluntary consent at its core (14):

1. Voluntary consent of the research participant is essential.
2. The experiment should yield important results that are good for society and are not otherwise producible.
3. The experiment should be based on prior animal experiments and knowledge that the results will justify the experiment.
4. The experiment must minimize harm to participants and have a favorable risk–benefit ratio.

Adoption of the Nuremberg Code was limited among medical researchers at the time, and there was no mechanism for enforcement.

Willowbrook Hepatitis Study

In 1956, Krugman and colleagues led a study of infectious hepatitis at the Willowbrook State School, a New York institution for children with mental retardation. The goal of the study was to investigate the natural history of infectious hepatitis, which the researchers claimed was highly prevalent at Willowbrook. The researchers deliberately infected the children with viral hepatitis and observed the natural history and response to immunoglobulin. The researchers claimed that they obtained informed consent from the children's parents and that they did not enroll children without parents or those who were wards of the state. Parents were also allowed to withdraw consent at any time. However, evidence suggests that parents were coerced into providing consent in exchange for admission of their children into the institution. Records also suggest that the managers of the institution manipulated the situation by creating a shortage of available residential space. Finally, the researchers attempted to justify inoculation of the participants by claiming that the prevalence of hepatitis was so high in the cohort that they were creating a controlled scenario, which they deemed inevitable given existing conditions at the institution (15–20). This case highlighted the risk of vulnerable populations being exploited for human subject research, and the concerns raised about the validity of an informed consent provided under undue pressure.

Declaration of Helsinki

In 1964, in response to the increasing prevalence of human subjects research, the World Medical Association published recommendations on ethical principles for physician–researchers, known as the Declaration of Helsinki (21). The guidelines highlighted fundamental differences between the therapeutic role played by treating physicians and the investigational role played by physician–researchers. The declaration has been amended several times, most recently in 2008 (22). In addition to the concepts of voluntary consent, favorable risk–benefit ratio, and sound study design, the statement emphasizes the need for independent ethical review of proposed research protocols.

The Belmont Report

In the wake of ethical controversies in biomedical research in the 1960s and 1970s (23), authorities in the United States took several steps to improve the standards of human subjects research. One major advancement was the National Research Act of 1974 and resulting formation of the National Commission for the Protection of Human Subjects of Biomedical and Behavioral Research. This commission issued the Belmont Report, a guidance document for human subjects research that distinguishes therapeutic medicine from research, identifies fundamental ethical principles for protecting research participants—respect for persons, beneficence, and justice—and describes how those principles should be applied (5).

ETHICAL PRINCIPLES

Respect for Persons

The ethical principle of respect for persons rests on both the concept of autonomy and the importance of protecting vulnerable persons. Autonomy is a person's ability to make decisions without inappropriate interference or obstruction. Autonomy also requires ensuring that the person's choices are respected unless they are harmful to others. The principle of respect for persons also acknowledges that not all persons are capable of self-determination, whether because of age, illness, intellectual or mental disability, or socioeconomic circumstances that limit one's liberty. For members of such vulnerable populations, appropriate respect and protection is required, and protections for these populations vary based on circumstance.

In the context of clinical research, respect for persons is the foundation of voluntary participation. Potential research participants must be allowed to provide voluntary informed consent before participating in a research study (5).

Beneficence

Beneficence is the obligation to maximize potential benefits and minimize potential harms. In clinical research, investigators must ensure that the study design is scientifically sound and minimizes risks for participants. In studies in which the aims of the research are to determine safety or efficacy of an intervention, an independent ethical review must determine whether the study can be implemented despite the potential risks. Moreover, investigators must establish adequate monitoring processes during the study to minimize risks and must exclude potential participants who are at inappropriately greater risk of harm (23).

Justice

This principle refers to the need to ensure that the costs and benefits of the research are distributed fairly. Vulnerable populations have at times borne the burden of participation in risky research—as summarized in the historical examples above—but often are the least likely to benefit from new therapeutic discoveries. More recent concerns about justice extend to our understanding of the benefits of clinical research in providing better data for medical decision making. For example, the US National Institutes of Health (NIH) requires the research funds to have adequate representation of traditionally underrepresented groups, such as women, children, and racial/ethnic minorities, when possible to help develop data about the external validity of clinical trial results for these populations.

PRACTICAL APPLICATIONS

To ensure that a clinical research study is ethical, investigators and regulatory authorities must consider every aspect of the study in light of the principles of autonomy, beneficence, and justice, in addition to any societal or cultural values and governmental regulations that may apply. Such assessment should be undertaken throughout hypothesis generation, study design, site selection, participant recruitment, and data analysis.

Informed Consent

Research participants should be enrolled in a study only voluntarily and after making an informed decision. Now a universally accepted standard of practice in clinical research, the informed consent process highlights the principle of respect of persons. In United States, this process is mandated by regulations for federally funded research (24). It includes disclosure of information to the potential participant, comprehension of that information by the participant, and voluntariness of the person's decision to participate (25). Informed consent is an ongoing process of communication and consent; the informed consent document is a record of this process.

Disclosure of Information
Researchers must disclose details about the research study to potential participants, including:

1. The objective and rationale of the study.
2. The duration of follow-up, the commitment required of the participant, and the procedures involved, with special attention to experimental procedures.
3. Clear descriptions of the risks of participation, potential benefits (including clear explanation of the role of placebos), and available therapeutic alternatives.

4. Full disclosure of the investigator's role in the study, especially if the investigator also provides clinical care for the potential participant.

Comprehension of Disclosed Information

A crucial component of the informed consent process is an adequate understanding by the potential participant of the information provided about the research. The information should be provided in clear, understandable language (including translation for non–English-speaking participants). Potential participants should have adequate time to consider the information and opportunities to ask questions of study personnel. Researchers should recognize that potential participants might have therapeutic misconceptions about the study; examples of especially vulnerable scenarios are when placebos are used, early-phase clinical research in oncology (26), and psychiatric research (27,28). Efforts to improve potential participants' understanding with the use of multimedia technology have yielded mixed results, but they may be particularly helpful in certain population, such as those with mental illness (29).

Obtaining Consent and Voluntariness

Informed consent should be obtained only after the potential participant is well informed and can make a voluntary judgment about participating. Potential participants should be under no undue influence or coercion. Financial incentives, limited access to healthcare for underprivileged populations, and fear of damaging the physician–patient relationship when the researcher is the usual care provider are some of the factors that can contribute to inappropriate influence on persons considering participation in research.

Informed Consent by Proxy Decision Makers

Some prospective participants might not be able to provide informed consent; examples include children, adults with diminished mental capacity, and patients in intensive care settings. If the research poses minimal harm (such as an observational study) or involves only noninvasive sample collection, informed consent by a legally authorized proxy can be straightforward. However, when experimental interventions are involved and they pose more than minimal harm, greater diligence is required. Respect must be shown for potential participant's prior interests and values when possible. Study design and scientific importance should be reviewed with extra scrutiny by the ethical review committee to ensure that the study cannot instead be performed in a population for whom direct informed consent is feasible. Research involving children should have the potential for direct benefit to the child. However, if such benefit does not exist, the study should not pose more than minimal harm and must be likely to generate results that will benefit others with a similar condition.

Exemption from Informed Consent

In rare situations or when obtaining informed consent is not feasible (such as due to time constraints), the requirement of informed consent might be waived. These situations usually arise in research concerning emergency or life-threatening situations, and when no proven or effective treatment option exists. Consent must be infeasible because of the timing of the intervention. In acute-care interventions, the short time window may preclude identification of a proxy. In such scenarios, a physician not involved in the research must agree that no other reasonable alternative exists.

Research that requires no intervention or interaction with the participant or use of the participant's identifiable private information also might be exempted from requirements for informed consent (24).

CASE VIGNETTE
IS INDIVIDUAL INFORMED CONSENT ALWAYS NEEDED FOR CLINICAL RESEARCH?

A clinical trial involving the testing of a blood substitute in trauma recently came under scrutiny. In the acute setting, obtaining informed consent is sometimes not feasible. In this case, a process called "community consent" was implemented, in which a series of community consultations was held to assess interest in the protocol. In addition, the researchers and sponsors developed an opt-out mechanism for the study by offering a blue armband to the community (30).

This protocol came under scrutiny from two different perspectives. First, a major newspaper announced that the sponsor had not published the negative results of a prior clinical trial of the product for a different indication. Can community consent be obtained if all of the available information about risks and benefits is not provided to the public? Second, a later meta-analysis of all previous trials of this type of blood substitute suggested statistically significant harm from this class of product (31). Should knowledge of the product class be considered in community consent?

Q: Is community consent an adequate substitute for individual informed consent for research when individual consent is not feasible? What would constitute an adequate community consent process?

Institutional Review Board

One important method for ensuring that research is ethically sound is to require review of the study by independent parties not directly involved in the research (25). This review includes assessments of the scientific validity of the study design and of the human subjects protections in the protocol, especially the consent process. Most research guidelines and regulations on ethics mandate that an institutional review board (IRB) or local ethics committee conduct an independent review. In the United States, establishment of IRBs is required by the National Research Act of 1974 and by Food and Drug Administration (FDA) regulations issued in 1981 (32).

IRBs have traditionally been decentralized, with local review committees most commonly associated with hospitals and academic centers involved in human subjects research. The usual composition of committees has included members from various backgrounds, including researchers, members of the general public, and members with legal and ethics expertise. The IRB reviews studies before their implementation, assessing the research protocol, informed consent forms, and any participant recruitment materials. The review is intended to ensure that the protocol will select appropriate participants and have a favorable risk–benefit ratio, and that the consent form presents the nature of the study and the commitment required of the participants clearly and accurately. The IRB reviews recruitment materials to prevent the use of misleading content. After an initial review, IRBs provide ongoing periodic oversight to assess protocol amendments, review changes to informed consent documents, and monitor unexpected events (32).

Challenges and Limitations of IRBs

The traditional approach to human subjects protection has recently drawn criticism, as research seems to have outstripped the original design of the review system and as the definition and types of research have expanded. IRBs were originally configured locally because clinical research typically involved single study sites. Today, although large clinical research programs can involve thousands of patients at hundreds of sites around the world, protocol review still is typically required at the local level, even when local scientific expertise may be lacking. In addition to duplication of review efforts, the system lacks dedicated resources for ongoing assessment of safety, given the tremendous workload such duplication generates at the sites. Reforms to address these concerns include the development of central IRB mechanisms for multicenter clinical trials and the development of data safety and monitoring boards to monitor trials on an ongoing basis.

Conflict of Interest

Many people are interested in the results of clinical research, including investigators who are concerned about career advancement, sponsors interested in drug approval and reimbursement, patients interested in access to new treatments, governments charged with holding down the costs of new technology, and the financial community interested in returns on investments in new medical technology. Those interested in the outcome of the study create the potential for conflicts of interest between actors in the system and the public interest in unbiased patient recruitment to clinical trials and unbiased reporting of research results (33).

In addition to financial conflicts of interest, physician–investigators must recognize the potential for conflicts in being both the physician responsible for providing clinical care and the research investigator focused on generating scientific knowledge. The two roles are different, a conflict that has the potential to jeopardize trust in a physician–patient relationship. The blurring of the two roles also can accentuate the "therapeutic misconception" by participants, as discussed earlier (34).

Management of conflicts of interest in clinical research has become a major challenge for the research and policy communities.

Types and Levels of Conflict of Interest

The conflict of interest associated with the greatest public concern involves financial incentives in research. These incentives can extend to financial arrangements for investigators, institutions, and research sponsors.

Patients expect physicians to be their advocates in clinical research and to provide independent evaluations of the merits of participating in the trial and when reporting trial results. Excessive financial incentives can compromise physicians' actual or perceived ability to fulfill these roles. As a result, many institutions have developed policies limiting the types of relationships between investigators and sponsors of clinical research and promoting transparency in reporting of relationships in publications, lectures, and patient care.

Institutions can have a conflict of interest when they have a financial stake in the technology being tested in clinical research at the site. Translational research can bring new clinical developments directly from the laboratory to patient care, but this also means that the institution can have an owner-ship interest in the technology. Managing institutional conflicts of interest can be more challenging than managing individual conflicts, because the institution sets policies for the conduct of clinical research and gover-nance of faculty investigators and supports the human subjects research review process.

Research sponsors can have significant financial incentives, especially smaller biotechnology or device firms studying single products, whose future can depend on the outcome of the study. Ensuring a mechanism for independence in design, implementation, and analysis can be critical in these circumstances, but this remains a sensitive issue with sponsors.

Although management of conflicts and disclosure remains the core components of policies to address conflicts of interests (35), disclosure of conflicts can have a counterintuitive result: investigators appearing to endorse clinical trials because they would be assumed not to have a finan-cial stake in a technology they did not consider to have merit (36).

Management of Conflict of Interest

In the current landscape of clinical research, complete avoidance of conflict of interest is simply impractical. However, disclosure of financial conflict of interest, independent oversight, and adequate training about relevant institutional policies with regard to conflict of interest provide mechanisms to safeguard the integrity of research and the objectivity of the findings. Generally, these policies describe types of relationships between investiga-tors and sponsors that are felt to be important to the development of the technology and scientific exchange but that are not seen as threats to the integrity of the scientific process. Relationships that involve financial investments, inventor ownership, or other types of equity (such as stock and stock options) generally receive the most scrutiny in these policies.

Disclosure of Conflict of Interest. During protocol review by IRBs and ethics committees, investigators are required to disclose financial conflicts of interest in accordance with institutional policies. Disclosure also can occur during or after the research to regulatory agencies such as the FDA and to peer-reviewed medical journals and professional scientific meetings. Most conflict-of-interest rules mandate disclosure by the principal investigators; these mandates might not extend to subinvestigators, who may be conducting most of recruitment and study procedures (34). Furthermore, IRBs lack the resources to provide ongoing oversight as financial arrangements between investigators and sponsors change during a study. Significant financial conflicts of interest also must be disclosed to potential research participants in a clear and succinct manner, and research personnel such as study coordinators, who are usually delegated with the responsibility of informed consent, must be familiar with information concerning investigators' financial relationships related to the study (37). The monetary threshold considered to represent a significant financial interest for disclosure differs across institutions and countries. In the United States, a regulation pertaining to conflicts of interest in biomedical research funded by the Public Health Service has set the threshold at $5,000. The ruling also requires certain financial conflicts of interest to be made publicly accessible, and that adequate training regarding conflicts of interest be conducted, before personnel engage in sponsored research (38).

Management of Disclosure. In cases where the potential secondary gain is significant, a management plan might be required to safeguard the integrity of the research. These types of situations frequently arise when a physician–inventor is testing a technology in which he or she retains an ownership interest or has equity in a company established to commercialize the invention. In scenarios where an investigator's secondary gain is perceived to compromise the objectivity of the research, limitations might be placed on the role and extent of decision making by the investigator in the study.

Academic institutions often appoint a standing conflict-of-interest committee to implement relevant policies. Institutional conflicts of interest might require a committee independent from the line of authority providing oversight of research administration (36).

Strategies to Minimize Potential Bias. The primary goal of clinical research is to produce generalizable knowledge that will contribute to better care and outcomes for society. This goal will be achieved only with unbiased dissemination of research findings. Several studies have reported potential bias in the publication of study results (39–41). One means of enhancing the integrity of the clinical research process is to establish independence between the trial's governance and sponsor. This can be done legally through site contracts (42), through clinical trial coordinating center agreements, and through journal publication policies mandating independent analysis and publication of results. ClinicalTrials. gov is a clinical trials registry established to reduce publication bias. Under the FDA Amendments Act of 2007, sponsors must now publish the results of clinical trials at ClinicalTrials.gov within 18 months after study completion.

CASE VIGNETTE

THE GELSINGER CASE—INDIVIDUAL AND INSTITUTIONAL CONFLICT OF INTERESTS

In 1999, a gene therapy study conducted at the University of Pennsylvania was brought to the attention of the national press with the death of an 18-year-old subject, Jesse Gelsinger. Gelsinger had a rare metabolic disorder that was controlled with special dietary restrictions and medication. He agreed to enroll in a Phase I study of gene therapy conducted by the Institute for Human Gene Therapy, aimed at eventually developing a new gene therapy for infants with a more severe form of the condition. Gelsinger was the eighteenth person enrolled in the protocol. He developed shock and acute respiratory distress syndrome after administration of the vector and died from complications of these conditions.

The university had recruited Dr. Jim Wilson to establish the institute as a signature program. Wilson was a leader in the field of gene therapy vectors and had established a biotechnology company to commercialize his inventions. The university established a strict conflict-of-interest management plan for Wilson years before the Gelsinger case, and the consent document fully disclosed the conflicts of interest for Wilson and the university. Despite these efforts, most of the scrutiny of Gelsinger's death revolved around the investigator and institutional conflicts of interest in this research (43–45).

Q: Should investigators with significant financial conflicts of interest, real or perceived, be allowed to take part in research from which they might benefit financially if a positive outcome is found? What about the institution where the study is being performed?

EMERGING ISSUES

Globalization of Clinical Research

Over the last few decades, clinical research has evolved from a local activity to a multicenter, multinational effort. Factors driving the globalization of clinical research include the high costs of clinical research in the United States and Western Europe, the potential to access more patients to participate in research, and the development of healthcare economies in emerging markets (46). Other factors include the potential for differing levels of regulation governing medical care and clinical research across markets.

The globalization of clinical research has been facilitated by dramatic changes in its conduct. Compared with the traditional model of academic collaboration in clinical research, most trials today are delegated to contract research organizations (CROs) (47). These organizations are usually commercial entities that provide services, including clinical research implementation and trials management, from early drug development (Phase I) to postapproval surveillance (Phase IV). This outsourcing of clinical research minimizes the need for pharmaceutical companies to maintain in-house clinical development staff and infrastructure for managing trials. The reliance on CROs has increased dramatically over the last decades, as reflected by the growth of CRO industry revenue, essentially replacing the traditional role of academic institutions in drug development (47).

Critics have highlighted some of the potential threats of this trend, mainly related to issues of accountability and research oversight. Because the primary responsibility is to pharmaceutical industry clients, emphasis is placed on completing the trials on time and within a competitive budget; less emphasis may be placed on the data collected in their totality. CROs are not typically independent of the sponsor and do not have the right to publish findings or approach regulatory bodies in the event of negative findings or even in the event of fraudulent research (47,48). Other concerns relate to high workforce turnover, which can compromise the effectiveness of trial monitoring and research integrity (47,49).

Although the benefit of closer international collaborations among clinical investigators should not be underestimated, several ethical concerns related to globalization of clinical research deserve special consideration. One question is whether the risks of clinical research are borne unfairly in markets unlikely to benefit from new therapeutic technologies. Although the life-sciences industries are targeting emerging market economies for growth, the bulk of the market for their products remains in developed economies. Given the sheer size of these markets, this phenomenon is likely to persist for some time. Thus, two basic questions are important. First, does the sponsor intend to provide access to the technology (if successfully developed) in the market where the research was conducted? Second, are the risks and benefits of clinical research borne proportionally by the intended markets for the technology?

Even if these questions are addressed, concerns remain about the implementation of clinical research in markets without a strong tradition of conducting it and without extensive experience in research ethics and human subject protections.

The ethical risks of this work are obvious, following directly from the ethical concerns raised at the beginning of this chapter. Payments to research subjects can easily pose serious ethical concerns when the payments exceed fair compensation and become an undue influence for those who are poor. In areas where healthcare resources are scarce, patients may be overtly or subconsciously coerced into agreeing to participate in a research study. Potential subjects' level of literacy and cultural context must be taken into consideration by investigators, especially during the process of informed consent. Societal norms also can compromise the notion of individual autonomy in providing voluntary informed consent, such as in paternalistic cultures in which decisions are made either by an elder or by the head of a household.

Before commencing a clinical trial in a community or population, investigators must assess whether the scientific question posed responds to the health needs and priorities of the population from which participants are being recruited. Based on the principle of justice, any benefits in terms of novel therapeutic products or scientific knowledge derived from the research should be made available to participants and the community. When conducting large multinational trials in middle- and low-income countries, investigators also must consider the appropriateness of using placebo controls, and whether clinical equipoise (50) truly exists when potential subjects are too poor to afford or have access to a reasonable level of "standard of care" (51,52). The latter issue can lead to questions about the external validity of clinical trial results for all markets.

Improving the understanding and training of investigators and research personnel in the design, conduct, and ethics of research is important to advance the quality and integrity of clinical research in developing countries (46). Increased transparency and accountability of the conduct and results of clinical trials also are vital in addressing some of the ethical issues arising from the globalization of human subjects research (46). Internationally adopted guidelines for ethical research, such as the ICH-GCP, can direct investigators (6). However, these guidelines are often subject to differing interpretations. Although laws and regulations may deter grossly unethical research, these vary from one country to another—they cannot be relied upon as adequate oversight without further investigation. Furthermore, in some low-income countries, limited oversight resource and potential corruption can further compromise the integrity of research.

In the longer term, continuing international collaborations among academic investigators and industry sponsors, ensuring appropriate investigator training in clinical research and human subjects protection before partici-pating in clinical research, and maintaining open and constructive dia-logue among stakeholders (including communities and regulatory authorities) will be essential to ensure the integrity of research that aims to translate into better healthcare delivery for all who have contributed to the process.

CASE VIGNETTE

THE GUATEMALA SEXUALLY TRANSMITTED DISEASE STUDY, 1946–1948

Recently, a grossly unethical study was uncovered by Dr. Susan Reverby of Wellesley College. The 1946–1948 study involved prisoners, institutionalized patients with mental disabilities, military personnel, and female sex workers in Guatemala. The study, led by Dr. John Cutler (a medical officer also involved in the Tuskegee study), was sponsored by the US National Institutes of Health. Study participants were intentionally inoculated with sexually transmitted dis-eases such as syphilis, gonorrhea, and chancroid. About 1500 subjects were involved, none of which appear to have provided valid consent. Some infected individuals received antimicrobial treatments, although most were inadequately treated (53,54).

In the wake of the discovery, the president of the United States issued an apology to the people and government of Guatemala. Independent inquiries were also commissioned to investigate the details surrounding the study.

Q: Discuss some of the main ethical violations committed by the researchers. Would similar incidents occur in the modern-day global clinical research environment? Are current regulations and guidelines adequate to safeguard vulnerable popula-tions in developing countries?

Research on Stored Tissue Samples

Many biomedical discoveries can be attributed to research using stored human tissue samples, especially in the fields of genetics and novel biomark-ers. The stability of DNA materials in nucleated cells allows researchers to use stored tissue samples obtained through a variety of means, either as part of medical care or in medical research. The landscape in genetic research also has shifted from the traditional individual team or institution focused on a specific, well-defined study to much larger analyses using samples stored in well-established biorepositories, often termed *biobank research*. Increas-ingly, concerns about the appropriate use of these samples challenge current ethical assumptions. The most contentious aspect relates to the need for informed consent and the nature of such consent (55,56). In the United States, research can be performed on existing tissue samples without explicit consent, provided that the samples have been de-identified and the person from whom the sample was taken can remain anonymous. This approach is based on the notion that such studies are no longer considered human subjects research as defined by federal regulation (1). In contrast, genetics research on existing tissue samples that are identifiable or linkable to the source, without prior informed consent, is generally considered unethical. The genetic information obtained from the research can have significant health, psychological, and financial ramifications. The ethical argument is that such research fails to respect individual autonomy (56).

The requirement of informed consent for tissue samples that are being collected prospectively remains a topic of debate among the scientific community and general public (57–60). If at the time of obtaining samples the intention is to perform research on them, even if only at some future date, the consensus practice is to obtain informed consent from the subject providing the sample (55). Nonetheless, no consensus exists about whether a (1) generic, unspecified consent indicating the intention to use the sample for research would suffice or (2) a more explicit consent, in which potential subjects might indicate for which type of research or even which disease conditions they allow the sample to be used, might be preferred. Some have even argued that subjects should be contacted to provide consent for each new study as it is being proposed, although most will agree with a one-time general consent (61).

Informed consent requires that subjects receive adequate information with regard to the risks and potential benefits of the research. However, when tissue samples are collected prospectively for future unspecified research use, a blanket consent may be viewed as inadequate. The potential risks to subjects in the context of biobank research are difficult to quantify, notwithstanding their tangibility or importance. On the contrary, some might also question whether a subject source (or even an heir) can lay claim to any potential benefit derived from research on the samples, such as profits derived from scientific patents. Precedent legal rulings have established that donors of biological specimens do not retain property rights in the samples collected (62). Although more empirical evidence might be required to guide researchers in developing an ethically acceptable approach, differences in preferences exist across various cultural and ethnic backgrounds (63–65). With the rapid developments in genomic research, consensus and sensible laws and regulations are needed to address these challenges.

CASE VIGNETTE
THE HAVASUPAI TRIBE CASE—CONSENT FOR STORED TISSUE SAMPLES RESEARCH

In 2004, the Havasupai Tribe in Arizona filed suit against the University of Arizona in relation to genetic research on stored blood samples. These samples were obtained by university researchers in 1990 as part of a diabetes study. The consent form at the time indicated that future research studying "the causes of behavioral/medical disorders" might be undertaken. The tribe members objected to studies using the stored blood samples that were perceived to involve socially stigmatizing conditions, such as studies of the genetic basis of schizophrenia. Both parties eventually agreed to an out-of-court settlement (58).

Q: What constitutes adequate informed consent for future research on stored tissue samples? Does the source of the sample (or family) have the right to determine the type of research that can be performed later in the future? How would incidents such as this affect the public trust in biomedical research?

SUMMARY

Clinical research is crucial to the advancement of biomedical science. The ethics of clinical research start from the core principles of autonomy, beneficence, and justice, an understanding that developed in the wake of tragedies in which these principles were ignored. Today's clinical research ethics extend well beyond these core concepts. These frameworks are not a static set of concepts and rules but require constant engagement to understand the appropriate applications of these core principles to current research environments.

REFERENCES

1. Office of the Assistant Secretary for Health. Human Subjects Research (45 CFR 46). http://www.hhs.gov/ohrp/humansubjects/guidance/. Accessed April 6, 2012.
2. Public Health Service, US Department of Health and Human Services. Instructions and Form Files for PHS 398. 2011. http://grants.nih.gov/grants/funding/phs398/phs398.html. Accessed April 6, 2012.
3. Office of Human Subjects Research, National Institutes of Health. Nuremberg Code. http://ohsr.od.nih.gov/guidelines/nuremberg.html. Accessed April 6, 2012.

4. Rickham PP. Human experimentation: code of ethics of the World Medical Association. Declaration of Helsinki. *Br Med J.* 1964;2(5402):177.

5. The National Commission for the Protection of Human Subjects of Biomedical and Behavioral Research. The Belmont Report. Ethical principles and guidelines for the protection of human subjects of research. 1979. http://ohsr.od.nih.gov/guidelines/belmont.html. Accessed April 6, 2012.

6. International Conference on Harmonisation of Technical Requirements for Registration of Pharmaceuticals for Human Use. E6(R1). Guideline for Good Clinical Practice. 1996. http://www.ich.org/fileadmin/Public_Web_Site/ICH_Products/Guidelines/Efficacy/E6_R1/Step4/E6_R1__Guideline.pdf. Accessed April 6, 2012.

7. Magiorkinis E, Beloukas A, Diamantis A. Scurvy: past, present and future. *Eur J Intern Med.* 2011;22(2):147-152.

8. Bean WB. Walter Reed: a biographical sketch. *Arch Intern Med.* 1974;134(5):871-877.

9. Jonsen AR. The ethics of research with human subjects: a short history. In: Jonsen AR, Veatch RM, Walters L, eds. *Source Book in Bioethics: A Documentary History.* Washington DC: Georgetown University Press; 1998.

10. Centers for Disease Control and Prevention. CDC—NCHHSTP—Tuskegee Study and Health Benefit Program. 2011. http://www.cdc.gov/tuskegee/index.html. Accessed April 6, 2012.

11. Jones JH, Tuskegee Institute. *Bad Blood: The Tuskegee Syphilis Experiment.* New York, NY: Maxwell McMillan International; 1993.

12. Katz J. The Nuremberg Code and the Nuremberg Trial. A reappraisal. *JAMA.* 1996;276(20):1662-1666.

13. Seidelman WE. Nuremberg lamentation: for the forgotten victims of medical science. *BMJ.* 1996;313(7070):1463-1467.

14. Nuremberg Military Tribunal. The Nuremberg Code. *JAMA.* 1996;276(20):1691.

15. Beecher HK. *Research and the Individual: Human Studies.* 1st ed. Boston, MA: Little, Brown; 1970.

16. Edsall G. Experiments at Willowbrook. *Lancet.* 1971;2(7715):95.

17. Goldby S. Experiments at the Willowbrook State School. *Lancet.* 1971;1(7702):749.

18. Krugman S. Experiments at the Willowbrook State School. *Lancet.* 1971;1(7706):966-967.

19. Pappworth MH. The Willowbrook experiments. *Lancet.* 1971;297(7710):1181.

20. Krugman S. The Willowbrook hepatitis studies revisited: ethical aspects. *Rev Infect Dis.* 1986;8(1):157-162.

21. Rits IA. Declaration of Helsinki: recommendations guiding doctors in clinical research. *World Med J.* 1964;11:281.

22. World Medical Association. WMA Declaration of Helsinki—Ethical Principles for Medical Research Involving Human Subjects. 2008. http://www.wma.net/en/30publications/10policies/b3/. Accessed April 6, 2012.

23. Beecher HK. Ethics and clinical research. *N Engl J Med.* 1966;274(24): 1354-1360.
24. Department of Health and Human Services. Protection of Human Subjects, Informed Consent and Waiver of Informed Consent Requirements in Certain Emergency Research. Final Rules (21CFR Part 50, et al., 45CFR Part 46). *Fed Regist.* 1996;61(192):51500-51533.
25. Emanuel EJ, Wendler D, Grady C. What makes clinical research ethical? *JAMA.* 2000;283(20):2701-2711.
26. Jansen LA, et al. Unrealistic optimism in early-phase oncology trials. *IRB.* 2011;33(1):1-8.
27. Appelbaum PS, Roth LH, Lidz C. The therapeutic misconception: informed consent in psychiatric research. *Int J Law Psychiatry.* 1982;5(3-4):319-329.
28. Appelbaum PS, Roth LH, Lidz CW, Benson P, Winslade W. False hopes and best data: consent to research and the therapeutic misconception. *Hastings Cent Rep.* 1987;17(2):20-24.
29. Flory J, Emanuel E. Interventions to improve research participants' understanding in informed consent for research: a systematic review. *JAMA.* 2004; 292(13):1593-1601.
30. Dalton R. Trauma trials leave ethicists uneasy. *Nature.* 2006;440(7083): 390-391.
31. Natanson C, Kern SJ, Lurie P, Banks SM, Wolfe SM. Cell-free hemoglobin-based blood substitutes and risk of myocardial infarction and death: a meta-analysis. *JAMA.* 2008;299(19):2304-2312.
32. Office of the Inspector General, Department of Health and Human Services. *Institutional Review Boards: Their Role in Reviewing Approved Research. Report OEI-01-97-00190.* Washington DC: Office of the Inspector General; 1998.
33. Thompson DF. Understanding financial conflicts of interest. *N Engl J Med.* 1993;329(8):573-576.
34. Morin K, et al. Managing conflicts of interest in the conduct of clinical trials. *JAMA.* 2002;287(1):78-84.
35. Weinfurt KP, et al. Effects of disclosing financial interests on participation in medical research: a randomized vignette trial. *Am Heart J.* 2008;156(4):689-697.
36. AAMC Task Force on Financial Conflicts of Interest. Protecting subjects, preserving trust, promoting progress II: principles and recommendations for oversight of an institution's financial interests in human subjects research. *Acad Med.* 2003;78(2):237-245.
37. Weinfurt KP, et al. Disclosure of financial relationships to participants in clinical research. *N Engl J Med.* 2009;361(9):916-921.
38. National Institutes of Health. NOT-OD-10-099: NIH Requests Comments on the Proposed Rule Applicable to Regulations on the Responsibility of Applicants for Promoting Objectivity in Research for which Public Health Service Funding is Sought and Responsible Prospective Contractors. 2010. http://grants.nih.gov/grants/guide/notice-files/NOT-OD-10-099.html. Accessed April 6, 2012.

39. Gibson L. GlaxoSmithKline to publish clinical trials after US lawsuit. *BMJ.* 2004;328(7455):1513.
40. Hrachovec JB, Mora M. Reporting of 6-month vs 12-month data in a clinical trial of celecoxib. *JAMA.* 2001;286(19):2398; author reply 2399-2400.
41. Kahn JO, Cherng DW, Mayer K, Murray H, Lagakos S. Evaluation of HIV-1 immunogen, an immunologic modifier, administered to patients infected with HIV having 300 to 549 × 10⁶/L CD4 cell counts: A randomized controlled trial. *JAMA.* 2000;284(17):2193-2202.
42. Schulman KA, et al. A national survey of provisions in clinical-trial agreements between medical schools and industry sponsors. *N Engl J Med.* 2002; 347(17):1335-1341.
43. Liang BA, Mackey T. Confronting conflict: addressing institutional conflicts of interest in academic medical centers. *Am J Law Med.* 2010;36(1):136-187.
44. Wilson RF. The death of Jesse Gelsinger: new evidence of the influence of money and prestige in human research. *Am J Law Med.* 2010;36(2-3):295-325.
45. Wilson JM. Lessons learned from the gene therapy trial for ornithine transcarbamylase deficiency. *Mol Genet Metab.* 2009;96(4):151-157.
46. Glickman SW, et al. Ethical and scientific implications of the globalization of clinical research. *N Engl J Med.* 2009;360(8):816-823.
47. Shuchman M. Commercializing clinical trials–risks and benefits of the CRO boom. *N Engl J Med.* 2007;357(14): 1365-1368.
48. Ross DB. The FDA and the case of Ketek. *N Engl J Med.* 2007;356(16): 1601-1604.
49. Wadman M. The quiet rise of the clinical contractor. *Nature.* 2006;441(7089): 22-23.
50. Freedman B. Equipoise and the ethics of clinical research. *N Engl J Med.* 1987;317(3):141-145.
51. Lurie P, Wolfe SM. Unethical trials of interventions to reduce perinatal transmission of the human immunodeficiency virus in developing countries. *N Engl J Med.* 1997;337(12):853-856.
52. Angell M. The ethics of clinical research in the Third World. *N Engl J Med.* 1997;337(12):847-849.
53. Department of Health and Human Services. Findings from a CDC Report on the 1946–1948 U.S. Public Health Service Sexually Transmitted Disease (STD) Inoculation Study. 2010. http://www.hhs.gov/1946inoculationstudy/findings.html. Accessed April 6, 2012.
54. Frieden TR, Collins FS. Intentional infection of vulnerable populations in 1946–1948: another tragic history lesson. *JAMA.* 2010;304(18):2063-2064.
55. Beskow LM, et al. Informed consent for population-based research involving genetics. *JAMA.* 2001;286(18):2315-2321.
56. Clayton EW, et al. Informed consent for genetic research on stored tissue samples. *JAMA.* 1995;274(22):1786-1792.

57. Gronowski AM, Moye J Jr, Wendler DS, Caplan AL, Christman M. The use of human tissues in research: what do we owe the research subjects? *Clin Chem.* 2011; 57(4):540-544.

58. Mello MM, Wolf LE. The Havasupai Indian tribe case–lessons for research involving stored biologic samples. *N Engl J Med.* 2010;363(3):204-207.

59. Wolf LE, Bouley TA, McCulloch CE. Genetic research with stored biological materials: ethics and practice. *IRB.* 2010;32(2):7-18.

60. Charo RA. Body of research–ownership and use of human tissue. *N Engl J Med.* 2006;355(15):1517-1519.

61. Wendler D. One-time general consent for research on biological samples: is it compatible with the health insurance portability and accountability act? *Arch Intern Med.* 2006;166(14):1449-1452.

62. Anon. *Moore v Regents of the University of California.* Available at: 51 Cal3d 120, 793 P2d 479, 271 Cal Rptr 146 (1990), cert denied, 499 US 936 (1991).

63. Wendler D, Emanuel E. The debate over research on stored biological samples: what do sources think? *Arch Intern Med.* 2002;162(13):1457-1462.

64. Pentz RD, Billot L, Wendler D. Research on stored biological samples: views of African American and White American cancer patients. *Am J Med Genet A.* 2006;140(7):733-739.

65. Fong M, Braun KL, Chang RM-L. Native Hawaiian preferences for informed consent and disclosure of results from genetic research. *J Cancer Educ.* 2006; 21(Suppl 1):S47-S52.

Principles of Clinical Experimentation

CHAPTER FIVE

Introduction to Clinical Experimentation

Robert Bigelow

EVIDENCE-BASED MEDICINE

The practice of medicine is an art, performed for the healing and reduction in suffering of individual patients. Doctors practice their art through skilled application of available medical knowledge. Before the scientific and technological advances made in the last century, medical knowledge belonged to a select few and was passed from teachers to students as if from parents to children (see the first point in the Hippocratic Oath) (1). Although much had been learned through careful observation of human anatomy and disease, empirical evidence on prognoses and treatment outcomes was limited. Rational treatment decisions could be made deductively or on the basis of accepted beliefs; however, the inability to obtain extensive empirical evidence left the value of many treatments unproven and poorly understood.

Modern medical researchers have applied the scientific method and taken advantage of advances in information technology to produce an ever-expanding body of evidence useful in medical decision making. The scientific method (construction of a hypothesis, design of an experiment, analysis of the data, and communication of the results) and the ability to collect and analyze large amounts of data enable researchers to study the comparative effects of different therapeutic approaches. Opinions on the best treatment for a specific condition are often considered to be hypotheses and tested in clinical studies. Application of statistical methods to data from large populations of patients provides the ability to estimate the average response to treatment, along with the variation in response among patients, and statistical models can be used to identify factors associated with better or poorer response.

The art of medicine has been greatly expanded through the use of evidence-based methods. Multidisciplinary teams design, implement, analyze, and interpret the clinical studies that collectively form the body of evidence. Modern scientific principles require study reports to be publicly available and subject to scrutiny, often leading to debate about the appropriate interpretation of the results. Assessment of the validity of study results requires consideration of important factors such as the method of data collection and cleaning, relevance of the study patients to those seen in actual practice, methods for minimization of bias, and even the motivation of the investigators. Views about the best treatment are routinely examined in light of shared evidence, which is used to develop guidelines to aid in medical decision making. Modern physicians must have the ability to understand and interpret evidence and to make appropriate changes in their practice in light of new findings.

The clinical perspective, focusing on a single patient, is now balanced by the statistical perspective, which makes inferences from populations. It is important to keep in mind that response to a therapy can vary from one patient to the next, and the results from a single patient therefore do not necessarily generalize to an entire group. For the same reason, results from a population do not accurately predict what will happen to each patient in the population. The goal of evidence-based medicine is to provide physicians with the best available information to make individual treatment decisions. This is accomplished by joining the clinical and statistical perspectives to identify approaches that produce the best outcomes for the most patients.

CLINICAL STUDIES AND CLINICAL TRIALS

A *clinical study* is any attempt to learn more about a disease and its manifestations, causes, or outcomes. Clinical studies range in size from small, such as descriptions of a few interesting cases, to large, including many thousands of patients. Larger studies involve construction of a database and the use of sophisticated statistical methods to analyze the data. *Retrospective studies* collect and analyze data from events that have already occurred. *Prospective studies* identify a population of subjects (cohort)

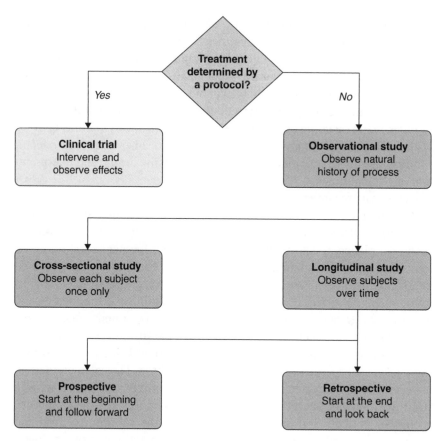

FIGURE 5–1. Types of clinical studies.

and follow them into the future from a specified time point, collecting data on events that occur as time passes. Our focus will be on a specific type of prospective study, the *clinical trial*, which has become the accepted best method for investigating the effects of medical treatments and the fundamental tool in the clinical development of new therapies (see Figure 5–1).

A clinical trial is a study in humans that evaluates the effects of a specific medical or health-related intervention. Clinical trials that produce the most reliable results have three important characteristics: (1) a quantifiable and relevant outcome, (2) the existence of a control group, and (3) treatment assignment determined by a protocol. This third characteristic implicitly requires a clinical trial to be prospective.

The quantifiable outcome in a clinical trial may be as simple as "Did the patient get better? 0 = no, 1 = yes." Or the outcome might involve a straightforward calculation such as "change in diastolic blood pressure from baseline after 2 weeks of treatment." It is not unusual for outcomes to be more complex, such as "time from randomization to cardiovascular death or hospitalization for cardiovascular causes, whichever occurs first."

In addition to being quantifiable, an outcome should also be a relevant measure of the severity or extent of the disease being studied, so that changes in the outcome are associated with changes in symptoms or signs of the disease. Relevancy of outcome measures, also known as *content validity*, should be a major consideration in both the design and interpretation of clinical trials.

The basis for inference from a clinical trial is the observed difference in the summarized outcome measure(s) between a group that received an experimental treatment and a group that received the control treatment, such as a placebo or no treatment at all. This difference is the observed *treatment effect*. The main analysis of a clinical trial reports the observed treatment effect for an outcome along with a statement about the probability of seeing an effect of similar or greater magnitude if the control and experimental treatments truly were not different. Treatment effect is most easily understood when it is represented by the difference between two means; however, it is quite common for the effect to be expressed as a ratio, such as the relative risk of a negative outcome. The calculation of an observed treatment effect can be somewhat complex; for example, in a stratified analysis, the effect is calculated separately for different subgroups of patients and then combined across the subgroups. Stratified analyses can produce more precise or accurate estimates of treatment effect and also provide the ability to test for homogeneity of the effect in different subgroups of patients. Commonly used stratification factors are sex, age, and race as well as known measures of risk observable at baseline. Even when study designs or analyses appear complicated, the treatment effect is fundamentally the difference between the experimental and control groups. Reliable estimation of the treatment effect requires a valid control group.

Assignment of treatment by a protocol reduces the chance that investigators might introduce bias by (consciously or subconsciously) selecting different types of patients for the experimental and control arms, thereby building in a difference between treatment arms that reflects factors unrelated to treatment. *Randomization* is the preferred method for avoiding bias in treatment assignment, because it assures that the treatment a patient will receive is determined by chance and is therefore unrelated to characteristics of the specific patient. Whenever possible it is advantageous to ensure that investigators and patients are unaware of which treatment is received. This technique, called *blinding*, makes it unlikely that treatment assignment for a new patient could be accurately predicted, and it also reduces the potential for bias in the reporting of measurements taken during the study.

The importance of requiring treatment assignment to be done by a protocol is seen in the example of an hypothetical retrospective study comparing myocardial infarction-free survival between patients who chose surgical intervention for single-vessel ischemic heart disease and patients who chose medical therapy. Comparisons between the surgical and medical groups might be confounded if patients who chose surgery tended to have a different baseline risk of negative outcome compared with patients who chose medical therapy. Statistical techniques could adjust the comparison to account for differences between the surgical and medical groups; however, the validity of the adjustments would depend on the completeness of information on baseline risk of the patients in the study. Stronger evidence on the relative efficacy of surgery and medical treatment could be obtained from a prospective study employing random assignment to treatment.

HYPOTHESIS TESTING

In the classical clinical trial, two treatments—control (C) and test (T)—are compared on the basis of a quantifiable outcome measure. We wish to know whether the test treatment is better than the control treatment, and the trial will have one of two conclusions. Either the test treatment will be proven to be better than the control (trial is positive) or it will not (trial is negative). Studies designed this way are called superiority trials, because the goal is to show that T is better than C. We assume that the means for groups C and T, μ_C and μ_T, represent the true averages of the outcome variable among all patients eligible to receive C or T. "Mean" in this context stands for a statistical measure of central tendency that summarizes the outcome in a group. The true treatment effect is $\Delta = \mu_T - \mu_C$, the difference between the average test group and control group outcomes.

To set up the mechanism for inference, we assume that there is no difference between the test and the control, that is, $\Delta = 0$. This is called the *null hypothesis*. If the null hypothesis is true, then we would expect that the results from the trial would produce an observed Δ approximately equal

TABLE 5–1		
Types of errors in hypothesis testing		
	Trial decision	
Truth	Positive (test better than control)	Negative (test not better than control)
Test better than control	True positive $(1 - \alpha)$	False negative Type II error (β)
Test not better than control	False positive Type I error (α)	True negative $(1 - \beta)$

to 0. In a positive trial, the observed Δ would be so different from 0 that we would not believe that the null hypothesis could be true. In this case, we would reject the null hypothesis and claim that there is indeed a treatment effect. If the observed Δ is not far enough from 0 to convince us that the treatments are different, then we have a negative trial, or a failure to reject the null hypothesis.

It is important to consider the possibility of making a wrong decision from a clinical trial. One kind of wrong decision would be made if we claimed that the test treatment was better than the control, when in fact it was not. This would be a *Type I error* or false positive. The other kind of wrong decision would be made if we claimed that the test was not better than the control, when in fact it really was. This would be a *Type II error* or false negative (Table 5–1). The sizes of Type I error (α) and Type II error (β) are specified in the design of the study and are important determinants of the sample size.

The ways that we control for Type I and II errors are conceptually different. This can be seen by examining how a test statistic determines whether a trial is positive or negative. A test statistic can be thought of as a ratio of the difference between the observed average outcomes $(\hat{\mu}_T - \hat{\mu}_C)$ in the test and control arms and the standard deviation, s_{diff}, of this difference. (For some types of data and statistical tests, more complicated formulations for the test statistic might be used.) A test statistic $(\hat{\mu}_T - \hat{\mu}_C)/s_{diff}$ is like a signal-to-noise ratio; the ratio is increased by a larger signal $(\hat{\mu}_T - \hat{\mu}_C)$ and decreased by greater noise (s_{diff}). *Statistical significance* is reported when the computed test statistic is so large that, if the test and control arms were not really different and we were to repeat our clinical trial many times, no more than $100 \times \alpha\%$ of the repeats would produce a test statistic as large as the one we observed. The P value is the computed probability of observing a test statistic at least as large as the one we observed, assuming the null hypothesis of no difference between the treatment arms. Statistical significance is claimed if the P value is less than the prespecified α. In most positive trials, the P value will be considerably lower than α. (Not to be confused with statistical significance is *clinical significance*, which assesses the apparent net benefit of a treatment for individual patients taking into account other factors such as the risk of adverse events or cost.)

Random assignment of patients to treatment plays an important role in the control of Type I error. It reduces the potential for bias in the treatment comparison by balancing prognostic factors between treatment groups. In addition, randomization introduces the element of chance necessary to interpret the P value as a probability statement.

The value of α is called the level of significance and is specified in the design of the clinical trial. It is conventional to set $\alpha = 0.05$, so that there is no more than a 1 in 20 chance of declaring a trial positive when in fact the treatments do not differ. Note that for a superiority trial, *two-sided statistical tests* are used, which means that a significant result can occur if either the test or control treatment is better. Thus, when $\alpha = 0.05$, the Type I error is really 0.025 (0.05/2), because cases in which the control treatment is significantly better than the test treatment do not count as positive trials.

To control Type II error (β), we consider a hypothetical nonzero difference between the test and control treatment arms ($\Delta_A = \mu_T - \mu_C$) and the anticipated variation in Δ_A (s_{diff} = standard deviation of Δ_A). The suggestion that $\Delta_A > 0$ is called the *alternative hypothesis*. With prespecified Type I error, Δ_A, and s_{diff}, the sample size is determined so that the probability of a nonpositive trial is no larger than β. The *power* of the trial is $1 - \beta$ and is the smallest probability of a positive trial, assuming that the true average difference between test and control treatment arms is at least Δ_A. In other words, Δ_A is the smallest detectable difference between treatment arms, assuming power of at least $1 - \beta$. It is important that Δ_A be large enough to represent a clinically meaningful treatment effect but not so large as to be unrealistic. The required sample size for a trial decreases with increasing Δ_A, and clinical trial designers can be tempted to choose an overly optimistic alternative hypothesis to reduce trial sample size (and cost). This could lead to an underpowered trial with a greatly reduced chance of finding a realistic treatment effect.

Power is conventionally chosen to be at least 0.8, so that Type II error is less than 0.2. In large trials involving major investments of time and

TABLE 5–2

Sample sizes per group in randomized trial comparing two means with two-sided t-test and Type I error = 0.05

	Ratio of magnitude of treatment effect to its standard deviation $\lvert \mu_T - \mu_C \rvert / s$				
	0.05	0.1	0.2	0.5	0.8
Power					
80%	6,285	1,575	395	65	26
90%	8,410	2,105	530	90	34

resources, sponsors may be unwilling to accept a 20% chance of failing to find a clinically meaningful difference and will enroll enough patients to provide power of 0.9 or higher. The additional costs of conducting a more powerful trial may be acceptable compared with the cost of doing another trial.

Without describing details of sample size calculation, it is enough to note that the sample sizes depend on the specified Type I and Type II error levels and on the ratio of the treatment effect to its standard deviation. Smaller Type I error, smaller Type II error, and smaller ratios require larger sample sizes. Table 5–2 shows the relationship between Δ_A/s and sample size. The possible effects of sample size on Type II error are shown in Table 5–3 (2).

TABLE 5–3

Relationship between sample size and likelihood of Type II error

Deaths	Randomized patients needed, assuming a 10% risk of death	Chance of Type II error[a]	Comments on sample size
0–50	<500	>0.9	Utterly inadequate
50–150	1,000	0.7–0.9	Probably inadequate
150–350	3,000	0.3–0.7	Possibly inadequate
350–650	6,000	0.1–0.3	Probably adequate
>650	10,000	<0.1	Adequate

Source: Reproduced, with permission from Yusuf S, Peto R, Lewis J, Collins R, Sleight P. Beta blockade during and after myocardial infarction: an overview of the randomized trials. *Prog Cardiovasc Dis.* 1985;27(5):335-371.
[a]Probability of failing to achieve $P < .01$ if risk reduction = 25%.

Published reports of clinical trials should contain descriptions of how the sample size was determined, including the sizes of the Type I and II errors, and the hypothetical magnitude of the difference in outcome between the test and control arms.

In practice, clinical trial designs can be more complex than the superiority design described above. Variations include evaluation of multiple treatment arms in the same trial, unequal sample sizes across treatment arms, intermediate tests to stop a trial or discontinue arms before completion, scheduled adjustments in sample size to maintain Type II error, and assessment of multiple outcome variables. Two examples of trials designed to show that treatment arms are *not* different are *equivalence trials* (designed to show that two treatments give similar results) and *noninferiority trials* (where the objective is to show that the test treatment is not worse than the control by more than a specified amount). Trials involving multiple tests of hypotheses should be carefully planned to ensure that Type I error is not inflated simply as a result of having more chances to "win."

The hypothesis-testing mechanism is useful when looking at a clinical trial as a binary decision (positive or negative) and might be most applicable to larger studies designed to demonstrate therapeutic efficacy. Many clinical trials, however, do not lead directly to a positive or negative decision. One example of a trial without a specific hypothesis test is a first-in-man study of a new drug candidate. The goal of such a trial is to observe side effects of the test treatment and learn whether it can be tolerated without major adverse events. Pharmacokinetic studies often do not have a specified hypothesis test, as the objective of these trials is to estimate variables related to the pharmacology of the treatment. Another example of a clinical trial without a formal hypothesis test is a comparison of side effect rates for two treatments given over a long term. Relevant outcome measures would be adverse event rates and time to discontinuation because of adverse events. From these types of trials, estimated treatment effects and confidence limits are useful in interpreting the results.

CLINICAL TRIALS IN DRUG DEVELOPMENT

Clinical development for potential new drugs is often viewed as having four phases (Table 5–4) (3,4). In Phase I, the drug is first introduced into humans, usually as a single dose or injection given to a small number of healthy subjects. Phase I studies of cancer drugs might be conducted in patients instead of healthy normal subjects, because potential therapies in

TABLE 5-4
Comparison of clinical trial phases

	Phase I	Phase II	Phase III	Phase IV
Objectives	Determine the metabolic and pharmacological actions and the maximally tolerated dose	Evaluate effectiveness, determine the short-term side effects, and identify common risks for a specific population and disease	Obtain additional information about the effectiveness on clinical outcomes and evaluate the overall risk–benefit ratio in a demographically diverse sample	Monitor ongoing safety in large populations and identify additional uses of the agent that might be approved by the FDA
Factors to be identified	• Bioavailability • Bioequivalence • Dose proportionality • Metabolism • Pharmacodynamics • Pharmacokinetics	• Bioavailability • Drug–disease interactions • Drug–drug interactions • Efficacy at various doses • Pharmacodynamics • Pharmacokinetics • Patient safety	• Drug–disease interactions • Drug–drug interactions • Dosage intervals • Risk–benefit information • Efficacy and safety for subgroups	• Epidemiological data • Efficacy and safety within large, diverse populations • Pharmacoeconomics
Data focus	• Vital signs • Plasma and serum levels • Adverse events	• Dose response and tolerance • Adverse events • Efficacy	• Laboratory data • Efficacy • Adverse events	• Efficacy • Pharmacoeconomics • Epidemiology • Adverse events

Design features	• Single, ascending dose tiers • Unblinded • Uncontrolled	• Placebo-controlled comparisons • Active-controlled comparisons • Well-defined entry criteria	• Randomized • Controlled • 2–3 treatment arms • Broader eligibility criteria	• Uncontrolled • Observational
Duration	Up to 1 month	Several months	Several years	Ongoing (following FDA approval)
Population	Healthy volunteers or individuals with the target disease (such as cancer or HIV)	Individuals with target disease	Individuals with target disease	Individuals with target disease, as well as new age groups, genders, etc.
Sample size	20–80	200–300	Hundreds to thousands	Thousands
Example	Study of a single dose of Drug X in normal subjects	Double-blind study evaluating safety and efficacy of Drug X vs. placebo in patients with hypertension	Study of Drug X vs. standard treatment in hypertension	Study of economic benefit of newly-approved Drug X vs. standard treatment for hypertension

Source: University of Pittsburgh Office of Clinical Research Health Sciences. Comparison of Clinical Trial Phases. 2002. http://www.clinicalresearch.pitt.edu/docs/comparison_of_clinical_trial_phases.pdf.

this therapeutic area can carry significant risks of toxicity. Study subjects are generally monitored closely for side effects or changes in clinical laboratory measurements. Blood samples collected at specified times after dosing are analyzed for drug concentrations to produce pharmacokinetic profiles describing the timing of uptake and elimination of the drug and any metabolites. These profiles are compared with profiles obtained from animal testing and used to select appropriate doses and regimens in subsequent studies. Drug half-life is particularly important, because longer half-lives can be associated with the possibility of accumulation and increased risk of side effects.

Later Phase I studies might further explore absorption, distribution, metabolism, and elimination (ADME) of the drug by evaluating multiple-dose regimens, bioavailability of oral forms, and comparison of pharmacokinetics between fed and fasting conditions. Phase I data combined across several studies might be used to evaluate the pharmacodynamics of the drug by analyzing associations between pharmacokinetic variables or blood concentrations and biological measures.

Early Phase I studies often employ dose-escalation designs, in which the first group of patients receives small doses and subsequent groups receive larger doses, after the safety of earlier doses is confirmed. For comparing two or more doses, a crossover design can be used to reduce the number of subjects needed for the study. In this design, each subject receives all of the doses, with an appropriate washout period between administrations. The order of receipt of doses is randomized. The crossover design produces a gain in efficiency, because test statistics comparing treatments use an estimate of within-subject variation in the denominator. Without the crossover, estimates of between-subject variation would be used in the denominator, generally producing less statistical power (see Chapter 6 for greater detail about Phase I studies).

Phase II studies begin to establish evidence of drug effect for its intended indication. Initial studies in Phase IIa test a range of doses in patients with the relevant condition. Dose-finding studies might be randomized comparisons of several different dose levels or involve a sequential dose-selection scheme, in which the choice of dose for future patients is guided by results in the patients previously evaluated. Randomized dose-finding studies are simpler to design and analyze; however, they may require larger sample sizes. Whenever possible, interim assessment plans are used to avoid unnecessary exposure of patients to inadequate or unsafe doses. Phase IIa should identify a "target" dose at which maximal efficacy (relative to safety) is expected to be observed. The Phase IIa target dose, or range of doses close to it, is tested in Phase IIb. Phase IIb trials usually are randomized and have sample sizes large enough to obtain more precise estimates of efficacy and adverse event rates.

An important goal of drug development is to show that the test treatment is statistically significantly better than the control with respect to outcome measures reflecting clinical benefit, such as survival, time to adverse outcome, disease symptom score, or functional status. Demonstration of clinical benefit can require large studies with extended follow-up, and sponsors are for the most part unwilling to commit necessary resources to large-scale trials without some evidence from Phase IIb that the drug will be effective. Thus, Phase IIb trials may evaluate *surrogate outcomes*, which are relatively easy to assess and generally require less follow-up than the true measures of clinical benefit. A good surrogate outcome should be associated with clinical benefit, and ideally there should be a biologically plausible argument explaining the association (4). Obtaining funding and institutional review board approval for a large clinical trial designed to show clinical benefit is easier if Phase II data have shown a positive effect of the treatment on a surrogate end point (see Chapter 7 for greater detail about Phase II studies).

Demonstration of clinical benefit is accomplished in Phase III by large, multicenter, randomized, controlled clinical trials, often including patients from multiple geographic regions. Regulatory approval typically requires "at least two adequate and well-controlled studies, each convincing on its own, to establish effectiveness" (5). Positive results from two trials can be viewed as squaring the Type I error (mistakenly approving the marketing of an ineffective new drug), which becomes 0.0025 (0.05 × 0.05). In some cases, overwhelming positive evidence from a large trial can be sufficient for approval, provided that the trial achieves a high degree of statistical significance for more than one important end point, a consistently positive treatment effect is observed in multiple subpopulations, and the results are so conclusive that randomizing patients to a control arm in a subsequent study may be considered unethical (5). The sample size in Phase III trials almost always provides >80% power to detect a clinically relevant treatment effect in the primary efficacy variable, and power >90% is not uncommon.

Phase III trials routinely include objectives of assessing treatment effect in subgroups, especially those determined by the age, race, or sex of the patients intended to receive the therapy. To provide more information about the utility of the new treatment, Phase III trial designers will often include secondary objectives measuring the effect of treatment on economic or quality-of-life variables. Phase III trials may contain substudies of specific populations who undergo additional testing, such as blood sampling for pharmacokinetic or -dynamic analysis. It has become common for biological samples from patients in Phase III trials to be collected and used in evaluation of unusual treatment effects (efficacy or adverse events) associated with specific genotypes.

Phase III trials can be expensive and time consuming. In addition to costs for patient care, substantial expenses are associated with staffing and administration at investigative sites. Manufacture, packaging, and distribution of study drugs also contribute to trial costs, especially when there are numerous investigational sites or drug supplies are limited. Activating and monitoring multiple investigative sites in different countries can require considerable travel and coordination by the clinical trial team. Despite advancements in electronic data collection, the cost of data recording and cleaning continues to be large. Most Phase III trials require ongoing data monitoring for safety and early evidence of efficacy, necessitating regular data cleaning.

Planning for Phase III usually starts early in the drug development process, so that large efficacy trials can be started quickly if Phase II studies appear to be positive. Despite an incentive to bring a new therapy quickly into Phase III, it is an advantage to have strong Phase II evidence indicating a high probability of success. Mean Phase III costs have been estimated to exceed those of Phases I and II by factors of 5.7 and 3.7, respectively (Table 5–5) (6), and it can be costly for a new therapy to fail late in development.

TABLE 5–5

Average out-of-pocket clinical period costs for investigational compounds (in millions of 2,000 dollars)[a]

Testing phase	Mean cost	Median cost	Standard deviation	N^b	Probability of entering phase (%)	Expected cost
Phase I	15.2	13.9	12.8	66	100	15.2
Phase II	23.5	17.0	22.1	53	71	16.7
Phase III	86.3	62.0	60.6	33	31.4	27.1
Long-term animal	5.2	3.1	4.8	20	31.4	1.6
Total						**60.6**

Source: Reproduced with permission, from DiMasi JA, Hansen RW, Grabowski HG. The price of innovation: new estimates of drug development costs. *J Health Econ.* 2003;22(2):151-185.
[a]All costs were deflated using the GDP Implicit Price Deflator. Weighted values were used in calculating means, medians, and standard deviations.
[b]Number of compounds with full cost data for the phase.

After a successful Phase III program and approval for use, a drug might undergo Phase IV testing to obtain further evidence regarding safety, such as effects of chronic treatment or adverse event profiles in subgroups. Phase IV studies designed to evaluate specific risks may be required by regulatory agencies as a condition of approval. Other objectives in Phase IV might include development of additional indications or pharmacoeconomic evaluation. Phase IV study designs vary widely, ranging from patient registries to controlled clinical trials (see Chapter 8 for greater detail about Phase III and IV studies).

SUMMARY

Application of the scientific method and technological advances in the collection and analysis of data have enabled researchers to study the effects of medical treatments on large populations, creating a body of evidence that can be used as a basis for medical decision making. Evidence-based medicine is supported by well-conducted clinical studies, designed and analyzed with specific hypotheses in mind, and can provide physicians global access to information on therapeutic effects, safety risks, and cost of available treatment options.

One special type of prospective study, the clinical trial, has emerged as the standard for testing and determining the effects of proposed treatments. Distinguishing characteristics of a clinical trial are a quantifiable and relevant outcome, the existence of a control group, and assignment of treatment based on a protocol. Clinical trials mirror the scientific method through specification of a hypothesis, design of an experiment to evaluate the hypothesis, collection and analysis of data, and reporting of results. Appropriate use of randomization and blinding help avoid biases in treatment comparisons and provide the mathematical framework to construct probability statements about comparative effects between two or more treatments. Because of the strength of evidence they provide, clinical trials have become the standard in development of new drugs and devices.

CASE STUDY

The chapters that follow discuss the Phase I–IV clinical development program for eptifibatide, a platelet glycoprotein IIb/IIIa inhibitor that prevents platelets from aggregating. The drug was first tested in human subjects in 1991, entered Phase II studies that same year, and began Phase III study in 1993. A New Drug Application (NDA) for marketing was submitted in April 1996, and the US Food and Drug Administration (FDA) granted approval for its use in patients with acute coronary syndromes in May 1998 (7). Two Phase IV studies were completed afterward: the Enhanced Suppression of the Platelet IIb/IIIa Receptor with Integrilin Therapy (ESPRIT) study in 2000 (8), and EARLY glycoprotein IIb/IIIa inhibition in non–ST-segment elevation Acute Coronary Syndrome (EARLY ACS) study in 2008 (9).

REFERENCES

1. National Library of Medicine, National Institutes of Health. Greek Medicine—The Hippocratic Oath. 2002. http://www.nlm.nih.gov/hmd/greek/greek_oath.html Accessed April 10, 2012.
2. Yusuf S, Peto R, Lewis J, Collins R, Sleight P. Beta blockade during and after myocardial infarction: an overview of the randomized trials. *Prog Cardiovasc Dis*. 1985;27(5):335-371.
3. University of Pittsburgh Office of Clinical Research Health Sciences. Comparison of Clinical Trial Phases. 2002. http://www.clinicalresearch.pitt.edu/docs/comparison_of_clinical_trial_phases.pdf. Accessed April 10, 2012.
4. Institute of Medicine. Evaluation of Biomarkers and Surrogate Endpoints in Chronic Disease. 2010. Available at: http://www.iom.edu/Reports/2010/Evaluation-of-Biomarkers-and-Surrogate-Endpoints-in-Chronic-Disease/Report-Brief-Evaluation-of-Biomarkers-and-Surrogate-Endpoints-in-Chronic-Disease.aspx [Accessed April 10, 2012].
5. Center for Drug Evaluation and Research, US Food and Drug Administration. Guidance for Industry: Providing Clinical Evidence of Effectiveness for Human Drugs and Biological Products. 1998. http://google2.fda.gov/search?q=cache: UPKx8ZoM4vAJ:www.fda.gov/downloads/Drugs/GuidanceComplianceRegulatoryInformation/Guidances/UCM078749.pdf+Providing+clinical+evidence+of+effectiveness+for+human+and+bio&client=FDAgov&site=FDAgov&lr=&proxystylesheet=FDAgov&output=xml_no_dtd&ie=UTF-8&access=p&oe=UTF-8. Accessed April 10, 2012.
6. DiMasi JA, Hansen RW, Grabowski HG. The price of innovation: new estimates of drug development costs. *J Health Econ*. 2003;22(2):151-185.

7. US Food and Drug Administration. Drug Approval Package: Integrilin (eptifi-batide) Injection. 1998. http://www.accessdata.fda.gov/drugsatfda_docs/nda/98/ 20718_Integrilin.cfm. Accessed April 10, 2012.

8. ESPRIT Investigators. Novel dosing regimen of eptifibatide in planned coro-nary stent implantation (ESPRIT): a randomised, placebo-controlled trial (erra-tum in *Lancet* 2001;357(9265):1370). *Lancet.* 2000;356(9247):2037-2044.

9. Giugliano RP, et al. Early versus delayed, provisional eptifibatide in acute coronary syndromes. *N Engl J Med.* 2009;360(21):2176-2190.

CHAPTER SIX

Phase I Trials: First in Human

*Kevin M. Watt, Karen Chiswell,
and Michael Cohen-Wolkowiez*

INTRODUCTION

T he development process for a new molecular entity (NME) in humans proceeds over several phases of clinical trials (I through III) before it can be approved for marketing by national regulatory authorities (Figure 6–1). Once regulatory approval has been obtained, after undergoing all required trials over many years, NMEs translate into drugs that are used to treat specific conditions.

The first step in human drug development involves Phase I or "first-in-human" studies. These trials are an exciting milestone in the drug development process, because this is the first time an investigational drug is given to humans. Before human testing occurs, preclinical (animal and laboratory) work establishes the preliminary safety profile of the NME and a starting dose for use in humans. At the end of the preclinical phase in the United States, the drug's developer submits an Investigational New Drug application (IND) to the US Food and Drug Administration (FDA) to obtain permission to begin human testing of the compound. The performance of an NME in Phase I trials helps determine its progression through the drug development process.

The primary goal of Phase I trials is to assess the safety of the NME in human subjects. In addition, the NME's pharmacokinetics ("what the body does to the drug") are evaluated to determine the most appropriate dose and dosing regimen in humans. Phase I studies also can explore the effects of different formulations, different exposure routes, giving the drug under fasting or fed conditions, and drug–drug interactions. Because safety and pharmacokinetics are primary objectives of Phase I trials, they are usually conducted in healthy volunteers (often adult men). This strategy limits

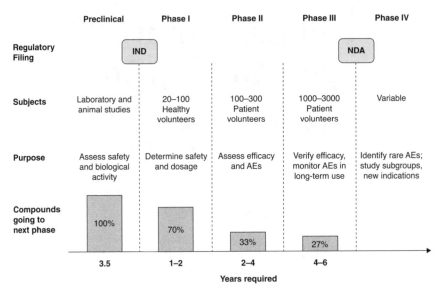

FIGURE 6–1. Drug development process. The process of bringing a drug to market is a stepwise progression. AEs, adverse events; IND, Investigational New Drug application; NDA, New Drug Application.

factors that can confound assessments of safety and pharmacokinetics, which are often present in patients with the disease of interest. However, in the case of significant toxicity concerns or a narrow therapeutic index of the NME, these trials may be conducted in actual patient populations.

The design of Phase I clinical trials varies according to the primary objective and can range from open-label to blinded, randomized trials. Phase I trials must show that an investigational agent is safe enough to be used in humans and must generate enough pharmacokinetic data to permit the design and conduct of Phase II trials. Description of pharmacodynamics ("what the drug does to the body") and early tests of efficacy can be secondary end points of Phase I trials, but the emphasis is on nontherapeutic objectives.

Phase I studies present several practical challenges to drug manufacturers. For example, the compound might not be available yet in the optimal formulation for the patient population of interest. Manufacturing the compound for these studies also can be very expensive because production of the NME has not been scaled up. Companies must balance the likelihood of the drug succeeding versus the resources required for the full-scale manufacturing process.

REQUIRED PRECLINICAL SAFETY EVALUATIONS

During the 1980s, scientists at DuPont began investigating a new class of antihypertensive agents that worked by antagonizing (blocking) the angiotensin II receptor. Early in vitro tests showed that adding angiotensin II to arterial tissue caused contraction of the artery, but adding angiotensin II and an experimental angiotensin II antagonist prevented contraction. After extensive engineering of the molecule to increase potency and obtain an orally active formulation, this candidate drug, dubbed DuP 753, was tested in rats and dogs (1–3). It was safe and efficacious in both species, but metabolism in rats created a highly active metabolite that increased the candidate drug's potency and prolonged its half-life. This metabolite was not created in dogs.

Before undergoing Phase I trials, an NME must go through extensive preclinical evaluations. These are done primarily in animal models that closely approximate the disease and the expected impact of the NME in humans. Animal models offer opportunities to elucidate drug mechanisms of action that would not be possible in human studies. For example, investigators studying DuP 753 hypothesized that the NME lowered the blood pressure by inhibiting the renin system. In one preclinical experiment, investigators removed both kidneys from anesthetized rats and noted that without the renin produced by the kidneys, DuP 753 did not reduce blood pressure (1). This finding confirmed the hypothesized mechanism of action of DuP 753; such a study could not have been ethically done in humans. Another important pharmacokinetic finding from preclinical studies of this NME was that production of a pharmacologically active metabolite was species dependent, occurring in rats but not in dogs (4,5). This finding raised the question of whether humans would produce such a metabolite, an important objective to define during Phase I human clinical testing. The presence of active metabolites could have safety, dosing, and efficacy implications.

Below are listed some of the preclinical studies that must be completed before an agent can be given to humans.

- Safety pharmacology in animals assessing the impact of the drug on vital functions (such as the cardiovascular system).

- Animal pharmacokinetic assessments, including evaluation of drug absorption, distribution, metabolism, and excretion (ADME).
- Single-dose (or dose-escalation) toxicity studies in two animal species.
- Repeated dose–toxicity studies in two animal species (one nonrodent) with duration as long as or longer than the proposed Phase I studies in humans. Additionally, the route of administration tested (oral, intravenous) should be the same as the proposed route of administration for humans.
- In vitro genotoxicity studies to assess mutagenicity.
- Reproductive toxicity studies to assess the impact of a drug on fetal development and female fertility, although this varies by region (5a):
  - United States—embryo-fetal development and female fertility studies do not have to be done before Phase I trials in women of childbearing potential, if the female subjects are carefully monitored, using appropriate contraception, and taking precautions to minimize risk of pregnancy.
  - European Union—a drug's impact on embryo-fetal development must be assessed before giving the drug to women of childbearing age. Studies assessing the impact on female fertility must be done before Phase III trials.
  - Japan—embryo-fetal development and female fertility studies must be done before giving the drug to women of childbearing age. These women must also be using appropriate contraception.

In addition to evaluating safety and elucidating mechanism of action in animal models, this study phase is used to estimate an initial starting dose in humans.

DETERMINATION OF THE MAXIMUM RECOMMENDED STARTING DOSE

The animal data showed DuP 753 to be a highly selective angiotensin II receptor antagonist. This agent, if brought to market, would be competing against angiotensin-converting enzyme (ACE) inhibitors. ACE inhibitors are not selective for ACE. They also act on the bradykinin and substance P systems, resulting in side effects, such as dry cough and angioneurotic edema, that often limit their tolerability. If DuP 753 was more selective, these side effects could be minimized, offering DuP 753 a competitive advantage over ACE inhibitors. Based on the selectivity of DuP 753 and its safety profile in animals, investigators established a maximum recommended starting dose (MRSD) of 40 mg (6).

Because the MRSD will be the dose tested in Phase I trials, it must be chosen carefully considering safety and trial efficiency. A conservative approach to implementing MRSD in humans (choosing a low dose) might lead to prolonged and expensive Phase I trials, testing several dosing levels to determine the most appropriate one. In contrast, an aggressive approach (choosing a high dose) can lead to excess toxicity. The MRSD is often extrapolated from preclinical data collected from animal models (Figure 6–2) (7).

An FDA Guidance for Industry (8) outlines an algorithm for estimating the MRSD in initial trials in adult healthy volunteers (Figure 6–3). The algorithm follows these steps:

1. No observed adverse effect levels (NOAELs) are extrapolated from data obtained from the most appropriate animal model. The NOAEL is determined from preclinical toxicology studies assessing overt toxicity, surrogate markers of toxicity, and exaggerated pharmacodynamic effects. The most appropriate animal model is usually the

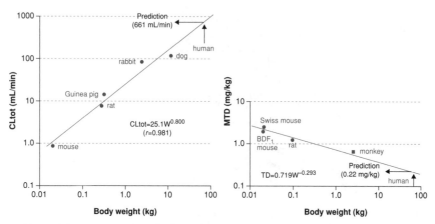

FIGURE 6–2. Example of allometric scaling of animal dose to human dose. Reproduced, with permission, from Peterson JK, Houghton PJ. Integrating pharmacology and in vivo cancer models in preclinical and clinical drug development. *Eur J Cancer.* 2004;40(6):837-844. CLtot, total clearance; MTD, maximum tolerated dose; TD, tolerated dose; W, weight.

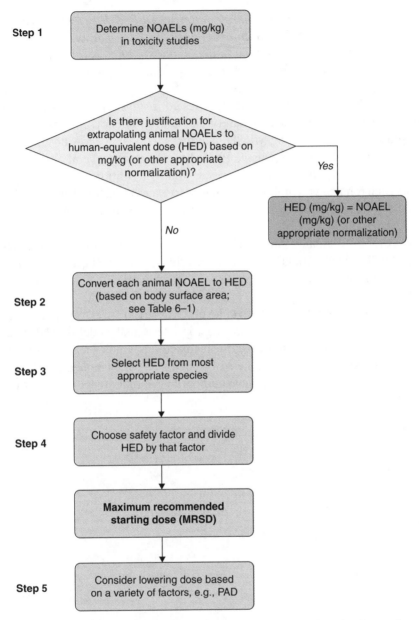

FIGURE 6–3. Selection of maximum recommended starting dose for drugs administered systemically to normal volunteers. NOAELs, no observed adverse effect (drug) levels; PAD, peripheral arterial disease. Reprinted from US Food and Drug Administration. Guidance for Industry on Estimating the Maximum Safe Starting Dose in Initial Clinical Trials for Therapeutics in Adult Healthy Volunteers; Availability. 2005. http:// www.fda.gov/downloads/Drugs/GuidanceComplianceRegulatoryInformation/ Guidances/UCM078932.pdf. Accessed April 11, 2012.

one most sensitive to the drug, but other factors can influence this choice, including variations in ADME among species and evidence that a particular animal model is most predictive of human toxicity.

2. NOAELs are then normalized and scaled to human-equivalent doses (HEDs) using body surface area-based allometry. The FDA has derived conversion factors for different species by which NOAELs can be multiplied to determine HEDs (Table 6–1) (8).

TABLE 6–1

Conversion of animal dose to human equivalent dose (HED) based on body surface area

Species	To convert animal dose (mg/kg) to dose in mg/m², multiply by k_m	To convert animal dose (mg/kg) to HED[a] (mg/kg) either	
		Divide animal dose by	Multiply animal dose by
Human	37	—	—
Child (20 kg)[b]	25	—	—
Mouse	3	12.3	0.08
Hamster	5	7.4	0.13
Rat	6	6.2	0.16
Ferret	7	5.3	0.19
Guinea pig	8	4.6	0.22
Rabbit	12	3.1	0.32
Dog	20	1.8	0.54
Primates			
Monkeys[c]	12	3.1	0.32
Marmoset	6	6.2	0.16
Squirrel monkey	7	5.3	0.19
Baboon	20	1.8	0.54
Micro-pig	27	1.4	0.73
Mini-pig	35	1.1	0.95

Source: Reprinted from US Food and Drug Administration. Guidance for Industry on Estimating the Maximum Safe Starting Dose in Initial Clinical Trials for Therapeutics in Adult Healthy Volunteers; Availability. 2005. http://www.fda.gov/downloads/Drugs/ GuidanceCompliance RegulatoryInformation/Guidances/UCM078932.pdf. Accessed April 11, 2012.
[a]Assumes a 60-kg human. For species not listed or for weights outside the standard ranges, HED can be calculated from the following formula: HED = animal dose in mg/kg × (animal weight in kg/human weight in kg)$^{0.33}$.
[b]This k_m value is provided for reference only, because healthy children will rarely be volunteers for Phase I trials.
[c]For example, cynomolgus, rhesus, and stumptail.

3. Extrapolation of animal data to humans is imperfect, so, after the HED is calculated, a safety factor is applied to incorporate a margin of error into the MRSD. Conventionally, the MRSD is calculated by dividing the HED by a safety factor of 10. In cases of severe or irreversible toxicity, narrow therapeutic index, novel therapeutic targets, or an animal model with limited ADME applicability to humans, a safety factor >10 may be applied. Conversely, a safety factor <10 might be applied for an NME that is a member of a well-described drug class with similar metabolism, toxicity, route, and frequency of administration. Drugs with limited, easily monitored, and reversible toxicity also might warrant a safety factor <10.

EXPERIMENTAL DESIGN

The move from preclinical to clinical trials signifies a significant increase in investment. The first Phase I trial of DuP 753 was designed in two stages, with Stage 1 being a single-dose study and Stage 2 being a multiple-dose study (6). During Stage 1, eight healthy volunteers were given either escalating oral doses of DuP 753 (2.5 mg, 5 mg, 10 mg, 20 mg, or 40 mg) or placebo. An exploratory, secondary pharmacodynamic component was added to the trial with administration of angiotensin I and blood pressure monitoring. Extensive clinical and laboratory safety evaluations were performed. Plasma drug levels were collected at specified times after each dose to determine the pharmacokinetics of DuP 753, and several neurohumoral variables (aldosterone, norepinephrine, angiotensin II) were measured as markers of drug effect.

The design of a Phase I trial depends on the type of drug and objective of the study. Because these early trials usually have a nontherapeutic objective (e.g., safety and pharmacokinetics), they are often conducted in healthy subjects. These subjects are volunteers and are often compensated for their participation. The number of subjects in Phase I studies varies by drug, but it is usually fewer than 30, and the sample size is often not determined through consideration of statistical power. Several factors contribute to the limited number of subjects enrolled in Phase I clinical trials: expected low variability in the healthy adult population, safety concerns, and the lack of medical benefit to study participants. Because subjects participating in Phase I trials do not have the disease of interest, it is challenging to evaluate drug effects in them. An antihypertensive drug given to a normotensive subject, for example, might have a minimal effect on blood pressure. The Phase I trial of DuP 753 was unusual in that the investigators artificially raised the blood pressure of healthy volunteers using intravenous angiotensin I, to collect data on efficacy as well as safety and pharmacokinetics.

In some cases, patients with the disease, rather than healthy volunteers, participate in Phase I trials. This is most common with investigational drugs that have a high risk of toxicity. In the field of oncology, new antineoplastic agents are often tested in patients who have advanced disease and few therapeutic options. These trials are often complicated by a more heterogeneous subject population but often have greater potential to show drug effects. These subjects are not usually compensated monetarily but hope to derive some clinical benefit from participating in the trial.

Surrogate markers of efficacy are often employed in early-phase trials, with good reason. Many chronic diseases can take years to affect health, making measurement of standard clinical endpoints (e.g., survival, functional status) impractical for small, early-phase trials. Elevated blood pressure is a well-described surrogate marker for cardiovascular disease that is easy to measure in a Phase I trial. Using surrogate markers such as blood pressure allows researchers to decide early in the drug development process whether an NME is likely to become an efficacious drug and thereby decreases the expense of late-phase studies of an ineffective drug. Additionally, in some cases these surrogate markers are accepted by regulatory agencies during the drug approval process, which reduces the lag time between conducting Phase I trials and bringing a drug to market.

The design of Phase I trials can range from open-label, single-arm studies to randomized, controlled, parallel designs with blinding. The appropriate study design depends on the study objectives. Most Phase I studies are open-label, but those incorporating pharmacodynamic or efficacy measures usually require blinding and inclusion of a placebo arm. When the objective is to determine the range of tolerable doses and the nature of adverse reactions with an agent, then a combined single-dose and dose-escalation study with a placebo arm is often used. For example, investigators in the DuP 753 trial assigned subjects to treatment versus placebo arms and conducted single- and multiple-dose escalation studies. With this design, they assessed the safety acutely and over time (multiple doses), described the pharmacokinetics of escalating doses, and described pharmacodynamics by comparing the drug arms with placebo. The investigators observed a significant decrease in aldosterone after administration of both DuP 753 and placebo. Without the placebo arm in this design, the drop in aldosterone likely would have been attributed to DuP 753.

DOSE ESCALATION

During Stage 2 of the Phase I trial of DuP 753, 29 healthy subjects were assigned (not randomized) in a single-blind fashion to one of five treatment groups (5 mg, 10 mg, 20 mg, 40 mg, or placebo). Subjects received study drug (or placebo) once daily for 8 days. In this case angiotensin II was given intravenously to elevate blood pressure, and blood pressure measurements were recorded. Clinical and laboratory safety was monitored closely. Pharmacokinetic samples were collected at specified intervals, and targets of drug effect (plasma renin activity, aldosterone, norepinephrine, and angiotensin II) were measured after each dose.

Once a starting dose has proven to be safe, the range of tolerated doses must be established. This step informs the steepness of the dose–toxicity response curve and is explored using a dose-escalation scheme. Two dose-escalation schemes are described below.

The first, the modified Fibonacci escalation scheme, is the most commonly employed escalation scheme in Phase I trials. Although it has a superb record of safety, it is often not the most efficient scheme. At low doses, when the risk of dose-limiting toxicity is less, dose escalation is rapid (Table 6–2) (9). As the dose and risk of toxicity increase, the rate of dose escalation decreases. In the modified Fibonacci escalation scheme, the escalation rate is predetermined and adjusted only if toxicity occurs.

The second method is an adaptive scheme that uses serum drug concentrations to adjust the dose in "real time" (Figure 6–4) (9a). This pharmacologically guided dose escalation (PGDE) method is based on the hypothesis that animal and human doses will show equal toxicity for equal drug exposure. Because drug effects depend primarily on the unbound component (i.e., exposure, that which is measured with serum concentrations), investigators can use serum concentration-associated toxicity data from animals and extrapolate to humans. Each increment of dose escalation

TABLE 6-2
Idealized modified Fibonacci search scheme approach to dose escalation in Phase I study

Starting drug dose (mg/m²)	Increase from previous dose (%)
2N	100
3.3N	67
5N	50
7N	40
12N	33
16N	33
etc.	33

N, original starting dose.
Source: Reproduced, with permission, from Goldsmith MA, Slavik M, Carter SK. Quantitative prediction of drug toxicity in humans from toxicology in small and large animals. *Cancer Res.* 1975;35(5):1354-1364.

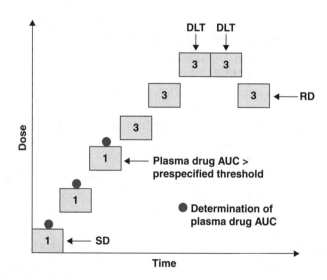

FIGURE 6–4. Pharmacokinetically guided dose escalation in Phase I trials. Each box represents a cohort comprising the indicated number of patients treated at a given dose level. DLT, dose-limiting toxicity; SD, starting dose; RD, recommended dose; AUC, area under the curve for drug concentration as a function of time. Reproduced, with permission, from Le Tourneau C, Lee JJ, Siu LL. Dose escalation methods in phase I cancer clinical trials. *J Natl Cancer Inst.* 2009;101(10):708–720.

is based on serum concentrations, which individualizes the escalation scheme. This approach limits toxicity by avoiding overdosing and maximizes effect by avoiding underdosing.

The DuP 753 Phase I trial did not employ a traditional dose-escalation scheme, although others did (10,11). Subjects in the Phase I study were given several doses ranging from 2.5 mg to 40 mg; however, the MRSD was 40 mg—the lower doses were given to better characterize the pharmacokinetics and pharmacodynamics of the compound.

CONCLUSION

Results from the Phase I trial of DuP 753 were promising. No adverse events were noted in any of the volunteers, and the pharmacokinetic/pharmacodynamic findings suggested that, as in rats, human metabolism of DuP 753 produced a highly active metabolite that increased both the potency (allowing for lower doses) and the half-life (allowing for once-daily dosing) of the drug. These results formed the basis for further trials that better characterized the mechanism of action and selectivity of the drug and ultimately led to Phase II and III trials, which showed efficacy on a large scale. The drug was renamed losartan (Cozaar®) and, as the first of a new class of antihypertensive agents, has become a multibillion-dollar drug.

The goal of Phase I trials is to establish the safety of an NME in humans. In addition, these trials aim to determine the minimum and maximum doses tolerated by humans and characterize the pharmacokinetics of the NME around this dose range. Data generated from Phase I trials are used to design future efficacy trials. As Phase I trials evolve, more emphasis is being placed on early efficacy measures that have traditionally been the domain of Phase II trials.

Both the European Medicines Agency (12) and FDA (13) now allow very low-dose ADME trials in humans (so-called Phase 0 or microdosing trials). Regulatory requirements for such trials are much lower than for traditional Phase I trials because the doses used are 1/100th of the starting dose for a Phase I trial, thus minimizing toxicity. The goal of Phase 0 trials is to better describe the pharmacokinetics of drugs in humans, so as to allow more efficient development of the most promising compounds.

However, safety assessments are limited in that the doses used in Phase 0 trials are much lower than the dose to be used in subsequent efficacy trials.

In response to the blurring of the boundaries between clinical phases of drug development, the International Conference on Harmonisation (ICH) released guidelines in which they instead describe the stages of drug development based on the objective: human pharmacology, therapeutic exploratory, therapeutic confirmatory, and therapeutic use (14). Although these changes can be confusing, they highlight the evolution of drug development and the diversity of approaches that can lead to development of safe and effective new drugs.

CASE STUDY: EPTIFIBATIDE

Eptifibatide is a synthetic cyclic heptapeptide derived in the late 1980s/early 1990s from a protein found in the venom of the southeastern pygmy rattlesnake (Sistrurus miliarius barbouri) *(15). It has a modified Lys-Gly-Asp (KGD) sequence and shows high affinity and specificity for the platelet glycoprotein IIb/IIIa integrin; reversible binding of eptifibatide to the integrin inhibits platelet aggregation and prevents thrombosis. The agent is highly potent, with a rapid onset of action and a short half-life (16), necessitating intravenous bolus and infusion dosing for prolonged antiplatelet effects.*

Eptifibatide was examined in 6 Phase I studies that comprised 69 healthy adults and 9 adults with moderate renal impairment (Table 6–3) (17). Half of the studies included administration of an intravenous bolus, followed by a continuous intravenous infusion for up to 24 hours. Bolus doses ranged from 20 to 90 mg/kg, whereas infusion rates ranged from 0.2 to 1.5 mg/kg/ min. Two initial studies were dose-escalation designs, with eptifibatide given as a continuous, 90-minute infusion of 0.2, 0.5, 1.0, or 1.5 mg/kg/min. Three of the studies explored the effects of various doses of eptifibatide when given with and without aspirin and/or heparin, because the target patient population for eptifibatide use (those undergoing percutaneous coronary intervention) would typically receive these therapies during and after their procedure.

TABLE 6–3
Phase I studies of eptifibatide (17)

Study	n	Population	Bolus dose	Infusion rate/duration	Other medications
91–001/001A	14	Adult men	—	0.2, 0.5, 1.0, or 1.5 μg/kg/min × 90 min	—
91–002/002X	28	Adult men	—	0.5 or 1.0 μg/kg/min × 90 min	Aspirin, heparin, or both
91–004	4	Adult men	—	0.5 μg/kg/min × 6 hours	—
	4	Adult men	—	0.5 μg/kg/min × 6 hours	Aspirin and heparin
91–006	4	Adult men	20 μg/kg	0.5 μg/kg/min × 6 hours	Heparin
	4	Adult men	40 μg/kg	1.0 μg/kg/min × 6 hours	Heparin
92–008	4	Postmenopausal women	90 μg/kg	1.0 μg/kg/min × 90 min	—
94–020	3	Adults with moderate renal impairment	70 μg/kg	—	—
	6	Adults with moderate renal impairment	50 μg/kg	0.35 μg/kg/min × 24 hours	—
	7	Normal renal function, age-matched	50 μg/kg	0.35 μg/kg/min × 24 hours	—
Total	**78**				

Safety was evaluated based on adverse events, laboratory abnormalities, electrocardiographic readings, the degree of access-site hematomas, and bleeding time during infusion and after study drug cessation. Pharmacodynamic effects were studied using ex vivo platelet aggregation assays, and the pharmacodynamic dose response was characterized. An important focus of the pharmacokinetic evaluation was half-life, which helped to inform the design of dosing regimens involving an initial bolus dose followed by continuous infusion of the drug.

The pharmacokinetics of eptifibatide were linear in the dose range of 0.5–1.5 μg/kg/min. The extent of drug binding to human plasma protein was about 25%. The plasma half-life was 0.59– 1.72 hours in the healthy men and a mean of 1.8 hours in the four healthy postmenopausal women.

Eptifibatide's effects on inhibition of platelet aggregation (IPA) were related to the dose and duration of infusion, with >90% IPA achieved with short infusions (90 minutes) of 1–1.5 μg/kg/min. Near-complete IPA was achieved by 4–6 hours during infusion of 0.5 μg/kg/min over 6 hours, although steady-state concentrations were not achieved during this period. This suggested that higher concentrations or doses might prolong the time needed to return to baseline but might not add to the drug's effectiveness. Neither aspirin nor heparin influenced eptifibatide's effects on IPA. Simplate bleeding time, however, was threefold higher with aspirin compared with baseline. Heparin and 0.5 μg/kg/min eptifibatide over 90 minutes had minimal effects on bleeding time, but eptifibatide infusions over 6 hours or of doses higher than 0.5 μg/kg/min were associated with a twofold increase in bleeding time compared with baseline. The combination of aspirin, heparin, and eptifibatide (0.5 μg/kg/min over 6 hours) was associated with a five- to sixfold increase in bleeding time.

After these Phase I investigations, investigators concluded that other than prolongation of bleeding time, eptifibatide appeared to be safe in humans with varying infusion rates, durations, and combinations studied. The effects on both platelet aggregation and bleeding time were readily reversible upon discontinuation of the infusion, with bleeding times returning toward baseline within 2 hours after termination, and platelet aggregation returning to baseline 4–6 hours after stopping the infusion.

THE ROLE OF TRANSLATIONAL MEDICINE IN DRUG DEVELOPMENT

The rate of approval of new drugs has fallen dramatically in the last 20 years, with only 110 new drugs approved between 2006 and 2010, down from 205 approved between 1996 and 2000 (18). Numerous bottlenecks exist in the drug-development process, including the ability to translate pre-clinical research into clinical trials. To overcome this limitation, the creation of early-phase clinical research units has emerged globally. These units break from a research model in which the various phases of drug development are done sequentially and in isolation from one another, to a paradigm employing an integrated team in which an iterative, often parallel, process flows from bench to bedside and back. These units apply novel systems biology and molecular medicine to early-phase trials to leverage greater volumes of data from early-phase trials. Incorporation of the -omic sciences (genomics, proteomics, and metabolomics), physiological assessments, advanced imaging techniques, and the identification and validation of biomarkers allows early-phase research units to expand upon the traditional Phase I pharmacokinetic safety trial. Through the integration of cutting-edge technology and flexible and efficient teams of researchers, early-phase units allow investigators to quickly and rationally determine whether a drug should proceed to Phase II trials.

REFERENCES

1. Wong PC, et al. Nonpeptide angiotensin II receptor antagonists. Studies with EXP9270 and DuP 753. *Hypertension*. 1990;15(6 Pt 2):823-834.
2. Wong PC, et al. Hypotensive action of DuP 753, an angiotensin II antagonist, in spontaneously hypertensive rats. Nonpeptide angiotensin II receptor antagonists: X. *Hypertension*. 1990;15(5):459-468.
3. Christ DD, et al. The pharmacokinetics and pharmacodynamics of the angiotensin II receptor antagonist losartan potassium (DuP 753/MK 954) in the dog. *J Pharmacol Exp Ther*. 1994;268(3):1199-1205.
4. Wong PC, Hart SD, Duncia JV, Timmermans PB. Nonpeptide angiotensin II receptor antagonists. Studies with DuP 753 and EXP3174 in dogs. *Eur J Pharmacol*. 1991;202(3):323-330.
5. Wong PC, et al. Nonpeptide angiotensin II receptor antagonists. XI. Pharmacology of EXP3174: an active metabolite of DuP 753, an orally active antihypertensive agent. *J Pharmacol Exp Ther*. 1990;255(1):211-217.

5a. International Conference on Harmonisation. ICH Topic M3 (R2), Non-Clinical Safety Studies for the Conduct of Human Clinical Trials and Marketing Authorization for Pharmaceuticals. London: European Medicines Agency, June 2009.

6. Christen Y, et al. Oral administration of DuP 753, a specific angiotensin II receptor antagonist, to normal male volunteers. Inhibition of pressor response to exogenous angiotensin I and II. *Circulation.* 1991;83(4):1333-1342.

7. Peterson JK, Houghton PJ. Integrating pharmacology and in vivo cancer models in preclinical and clinical drug development. *Eur J Cancer.* 2004;40 (6):837-844.

8. US Food and Drug Administration. Guidance for Industry on Estimating the Maximum Safe Starting Dose in Initial Clinical Trials for Therapeutics in Adult Healthy Volunteers; Availability. 2005. http://www.fda.gov/downloads/Drugs/GuidanceComplianceRegulatoryInformation/Guidances/UCM078932. pdf. Accessed April 11, 2012.

9. Goldsmith MA, Slavik M, Carter SK. Quantitative prediction of drug toxicity in humans from toxicology in small and large animals. *Cancer Res.* 1975;35 (5):1354-1364.

9a. Le Tourneau C, Lee JJ, Siu LL. Dose escalation methods in phase I cancer clinical trials. *J Natl Cancer Inst.* 2009;101(10):708-720.

10. Munafo A, et al. Drug concentration response relationships in normal volunteers after oral administration of losartan, an angiotensin II receptor antagonist. *Clin Pharmacol Ther.* 1992;51(5):513-521.

11. Ohtawa M, Takayama F, Saitoh K, Yoshinaga T, Nakashima M. Pharmacokinetics and biochemical efficacy after single and multiple oral administration of losartan, an orally active nonpeptide angiotensin II receptor antagonist, in humans. *Br J Clin Pharmacol.* 1993;35(3):290-297.

12. European Medicines Agency. ICH Topic M 3 (R2): Non-Clinical Safety Studies for the Conduct of Human Clinical Trials and Marketing Authorization for Pharmaceuticals. CPMP/ICH/286/95. 2008. http://www.ema.europa. eu/ema/pages/includes/document/open_document.jsp?webContentId= WC500002941. Accessed April 16, 2012.

13. Center for Drug Evaluation and Research, US Food and Drug Administration. Guidance for Industry, Investigators, and Reviewers: Exploratory IND Studies. 2006. http://www.fda.gov/downloads/Drugs/GuidanceCompliance RegulatoryInformation/Guidances/UCM078933.pdf. Accessed April 16, 2012.

14. International Conference on Harmonisation of Technical Requirements for Registration of Pharmaceuticals for Human Use. E8. General Considerations for Clinical Trials. 1997. http://www.ich.org/products/guidelines/efficacy/efficacy-single/article/general-considerations-for-clinical-trials.html. Accessed April 16, 2012.

15. Scarborough RM, et al. Barbourin. A GPIIb-IIIa-specific integrin antagonist from the venom of Sistrurus m. barbouri. *J Biol Chem.* 1991;266(15): 9359-9362.

16. Phillips DR, Scarborough RM. Clinical pharmacology of eptifibatide. *Am J Cardiol*. 1997;80(4A):11B-20B.
17. Center for Drug Evaluation and Research, US Food and Drug Administration. Clinical Pharmacology/Biopharmaceutics Review. NDA 20–718. 1998. http://www.accessdata.fda.gov/drugsatfda_docs/nda/2001/20–718_Integrilin_biopharmr.pdf. Accessed April 16, 2012.
18. Mullard A. 2010 FDA drug approvals. *Nat Rev Drug Discov*. 2011;10(2): 82-85.

CHAPTER SEVEN

Phase II
Clinical Trials

Jeffrey T. Guptill and Karen Chiswell

INTRODUCTION

Following preclinical and first-in-human (Phase I) studies, an investigational drug or device is studied in subjects who have the disorder of interest. This phase of development is commonly called Phase II or exploratory therapeutic development. Major goals of Phase II studies are to support the proof of concept or proof of mechanism identified during preclinical development and to show evidence of efficacy that will support future confirmatory trials (Table 7–1). Other objectives include defining the target population, exploring the pharmacodynamic relationship between dosing regimens and the effects on disease, determining the proposed dosing regimen for future trials, and providing preliminary estimates of drug effect to be used in calculating sample sizes for Phase III trials.

The objectives of Phase II support a critical "go/no-go" decision with regard to further clinical development. Sponsors usually prefer to abandon ineffective drugs early rather than waiting for resource- and time-intensive Phase III trials to tell them that the therapeutic has failed. Proof of mechanism, proof of concept, and identification of a therapeutic dose range and regimen are desired as early as possible. An inability to define any of these delays the clinical development program and may ultimately "kill" the therapeutic. Thus, the Phase II program should support the predefined goals of the clinical development plan and the target product labeling. The critical decision points and the criteria for the go/no-go decision are often determined as part of the clinical development plan.

TABLE 7–1
Objectives of Phase II clinical development
• Show proof of concept, proof of mechanism • Obtain an efficacy signal • Explore pharmacokinetic/pharmacodynamic relationships • Identify dose regimen(s) for further study • Define the target population • Evaluate short-term safety

Dividing the clinical drug development process into numbered phases implies a linear progression; in fact, Phase II activities regularly occur while pivotal Phase III trials are active. Such overlap with other phases is not uncommon, particularly when a drug is evaluated in understudied subgroups within a target population. In some cases, a well-designed Phase II dose–response study can serve as one of the pivotal studies to be submitted to regulatory agencies for marketing approval.

CHARACTERISTICS OF PHASE II STUDIES

Phase II trials are generally short, enroll a relatively small number of subjects (up to 300), and often use surrogate rather than clinical end points (1,2). Phase II is sometimes divided into Phase IIa and Phase IIb (or early and late Phase II) to indicate the shifting goals of this phase over time. Phase I and IIa activities collectively represent "completion of clinical trials that provide data on the relationship of dosing and response for the particular intended use (including trials on the impact of dose ranging on safety, biomarkers, and proof of concept)" (3). In contrast to Phase IIa trials, late exploratory therapeutic trials tend to last longer, have larger sample sizes, and place greater emphasis on the clinical efficacy end points to be used in Phase III.

Phase II seeks to define the optimum loading and maintenance doses, dosing interval, and treatment duration in humans. Investigators commonly give multiple doses of the study drug against a comparator or placebo, and a dose–response curve is generated that describes the pharmacodynamic relationship between the dosing regimen and effect. The shape of the dose–response curve, tolerability at varying doses, maximum tolerated dose,

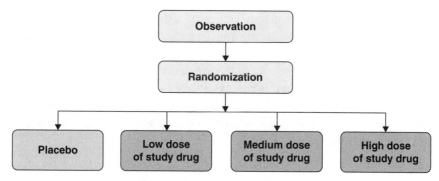

FIGURE 7–1. Illustration of a randomized, parallel-group, placebo-controlled clinical trial. After a period of observation, subjects are randomized to receive various dose regimens of the study drug or placebo.

minimum dose achieving maximum desired effect, and the safety and efficacy of varying drug doses are studied. The study drug also can be given with commonly coadministered medications to explore drug–drug interactions. Information from studies of other compounds with a similar mechanism of action can be useful—for example, to help select a surrogate end point or a study population.

The drug doses incorporated into early Phase II trials are determined from preclinical safety and effectiveness data and Phase I pharmacokinetic studies. A parallel-group design with several fixed doses is common (Figure 7–1). There are often several treatment groups with different dosing regimens, and each enrolled subject is assigned to one of the treatment groups. Late Phase II trials select dose regimens that appear optimal from earlier studies, but they can also include additional exploratory dosing schemes.

In some cases, an adaptive study design is used (4), in which scheduled interim data analyses drive predetermined changes in the trial's conduct, such as shifting enrollment to treatment subgroups that are more promising, or eliminating treatment groups (e.g., a failing dose arm) altogether. To improve the chances of success in Phase III, a potentially safe and effective dose regimen in the appropriate patient population must be identified during Phase II with as much certainty as possible.

Additional studies might be required later during development to support the use of the study drug in subpopulations such as elderly persons or patients with renal dysfunction or hepatic impairment. Emphasis has increased recently on including special populations earlier in clinical development (e.g., during Phase II) (5,6). It also might be relevant to evaluate drug dosing in various stages of a disease, such as early after disease onset versus late stage, and in patients with different disease severities.

Interest is increasing regarding the use of drug modeling and simulation to assist in dose finding. In this context, Phase I and II pharmacokinetic and pharmacodynamic data are used to simulate dosing in humans, hopefully leading to earlier identification of an effective dosing strategy and reduced development time.

EFFECT OF THE GLOBALIZATION OF DRUG DEVELOPMENT ON PHASE II

Although in the past the pharmaceutical industry relied on a small number of domestic sites for Phase II studies, drug development has increasingly become a global enterprise. More clinical trials are being conducted outside the United States, and pharmaceutical companies might outsource many roles within a study to international contract research organizations (CROs) or academic research organizations (AROs) (7). Studying drugs outside the United States may confer several advantages to manufacturers, including reduced costs, faster enrollment, and fewer local regulatory hurdles. In addition, drug metabolism and drug effects can differ by region and genetic makeup; if drugs are to be marketed in diverse populations, it is often necessary to study them in different geographic regions or in different genetic populations. These factors, together with potentially large increases in markets in developing countries, have led to more Phase II studies being conducted outside the United States. Even small Phase II trials now commonly involve multiple centers and international collaborators. Despite the potential rewards, this trend increases the complexity of trials in many areas, including regulatory agency interactions, institutional review boards (IRBs), site monitoring, data management, and ensuring data quality, drug supply, safety monitoring, and communication among investigators, trial sponsors, contractors, etc. As an example, an international Phase II study that includes multiple timed blood sampling for pharmacokinetic measurements may require detailed, multilingual instructions for obtaining the samples, as well as complicated logistics for shipping them to a central laboratory in another country for processing and storage until the assays are completed. An in-depth discussion of international research can be found in Chapter 4.

PHASE II EPTIFIBATIDE STUDIES

The story of eptifibatide will serve to exemplify the concepts discussed above.

Several inhibitors of platelet aggregation have been developed that have the potential to prevent thrombotic events, such as myocardial infarction (MI) and stroke (8). Eptifibatide is a synthetic platelet integrin glycoprotein IIb/IIIa inhibitor that blocks ADP-induced platelet aggregation (9). After Phase I studies showed no immediate safety risks, eptifibatide was evaluated in Phase II trials. During this phase, the drug was given to subjects with coronary artery disease.

Five of the eptifibatide trials (Table 7–2) (10–14) illustrate several characteristics of Phase II studies:

- Relatively small sample sizes resulted in insufficient power to show statistically significant differences between treatment groups with respect to clinical efficacy end points.

- Although trials were relatively small, they were all conducted at multiple centers.

- Studies had relatively short follow-up periods for clinical and safety end points (as short as 24 hours and as long as 30 days).

- All studies included more than one eptifibatide arm to compare different dosing regimens. Regimens could differ in initial bolus dose, continuous infusion dose, and/or continuous infusion duration.

- Different trials enrolled patients with different disease states—e.g., patients scheduled for elective coronary intervention, patients receiving thrombolytic therapy for acute MI, and those with unstable angina—to explore the relative safety and efficacy of the drug in different disorders and identify the most promising environment for Phase III studies.

- All studies collected data on inhibition of platelet aggregation, and a major focus of analysis was to identify a dosing regimen that both provided acceptable levels of platelet aggregation inhibition for an acceptable duration and showed rapid reversibility of effects after termination of eptifibatide infusion. Of interest, the ex vivo platelet aggregation assay in the Integrilin (eptifibatide) to Minimize Platelet Aggregation and Coronary Thrombosis (IMPACT) series of studies used sodium citrate as an anticoagulant

TABLE 7–2
Characteristics of five Phase II placebo-controlled trials of eptifibatide[a]

Study (Enrollment)	Patients	n	Study design	Eptifibatide arms[b]	Concomitant medications	Efficacy end points	PD end points	PK measured?
IMPACT (1992–1993) (10)	Scheduled elective CBA or DCA	150 at 11 sites	Randomized, double-blind, parallel-group	90/1.0/4 90/1.0/12	Aspirin, heparin	30-day clinical composite[c]	Substudy: IPA, simplate bleeding times	No
IMPACT High-Low (1993) (11)	Elective CBA	73 at 3 sites	Randomized; double- and single-blind components; sequential groups	180/1.0/18–24 135/0.5/18–24 90/0.75/18–24 135/0.75/18–24	Aspirin, heparin	Procedural success[d]; in-hospital clinical composite[e]	IPA[f]; simplate bleeding times	No
IMPACT-AMI (1993–1995) (12)	Thrombolysis for acute MI	180 at 13 sites	Randomized; open-label and double-blind components; sequential groups with dose escalation	36/0.2/24 72/0.4/24 108/0.6/24[g] 135/0.75/24[g] 135/0.75/24 180/0.75/24 180/0.75/24[h]	Aspirin, heparin, accelerated alteplase	TIMI Grade 3 flow in IRA 90 min after start of thrombolysis, ST-segment recovery, in-hospital clinical composite[i]	IPA[i]	No

Study	Condition	N at sites	Design	Eptifibatide dose[b]	Concomitant therapy	Endpoints	Substudy	Double-blind
IMPACT-USA (1995–1997) (13)	Unstable angina	227 at 15 sites	Randomized, double-blind, parallel-group, multicenter	45/0.5/24–72 90/1.0/24–72	Heparin, aspirin (randomized and after study drug stopped)	Number/duration of ischemic ECG episodes in 24 h and after drug stopped; number/duration of symptomatic ischemic episodes; in-hospital clinical composite[j]	Substudy: IPA[f], simplate bleeding times	No
PRIDE (1996–1997) (14)	Elective coronary intervention	127 at 14 sites	Randomized, double-blind, parallel-group	135/0.75/2–24 180/2.0/20–24 250/3.0/20–24	Heparin	30-day ischemic cardiovascular events	IPA[k], GP IIb/IIIa receptor occupancy	Yes

[a]These are five of the several Phase II studies of eptifibatide. All studies assessed bleeding as a safety focus.

[b]Eptifibatide arms shown as (bolus dose as (bolus dose in μg/kg)/(infusion dose in μg/kg)/(infusion duration in hours).

[c]Death (all-cause), myocardial infarction (MI), urgent or emergency coronary intervention, stent implantation, or coronary artery bypass surgery (CABG) for ischemia or threatened closure. CBA, coronary balloon angioplasty; DCA, directional coronary atherectomy.

[d]Residual stenosis <50% in the treated vessel as determined visually by the operator.

[e]Death, MI, CABG, repeat intervention (catheterization and/or angioplasty), or recurrent ischemia.

[f]Ex vivo inhibition of activated platelet aggregation (IPA) in citrate-anticoagulated blood. ECG, electrocardiographic.

[g]No heparin bolus.

[h]Double-blind.

[i]Death, reinfarction, stroke, revascularization, new heart failure, or pulmonary edema. TIMI, Thrombolysis In Myocardial Infarction; IRA, infarct-related artery.

[j]Death, MI, or refractory ischemia.

[k]Ex vivo IPA in D-phenylalanyl-L-prolyl-L-arginine chloromethylketone (PPACK)- and citrate-anticoagulated blood. GP, glycoprotein.

(10–13), which was later shown to overestimate the aggregation inhibition and receptor occupancy effects of eptifibatide (15). The Platelet Aggregation and Receptor Occupancy with Integrilin—a Dynamic Evaluation (PRIDE) study (14) used an anticoagulant that does not affect platelet function (D-phenylalanyl-L-prolyl-L-arginine chloromethylketone; PPACK), and it compared estimates of inhibition and receptor occupancy using PPACK with those obtained from the same blood samples but using sodium citrate as the anticoagulant.

- The Phase II studies were used to inform decisions about proceeding to Phase III and, if so, the dose regimens to be used:
  - The IMPACT and IMPACT High–Low studies were used to decide the doses to be used in the Phase III IMPACT-II study.
  - These same studies, along with the IMPACT-USA study, informed the dose regimens used in the Phase III Platelet Glycoprotein IIb/IIIa in Unstable Angina: Receptor Suppression Using Integrilin Therapy (PURSUIT) trial (16).
  - The last Phase II study conducted, PRIDE, studied rates of eptifibatide infusion that were higher than had been used in all of these earlier Phase II and III studies. One of the dose regimens used in the PRIDE study had been used in the IMPACT-II trial (17), and another had been used in PURSUIT (16). The goal of the PRIDE study was to fill in gaps in knowledge regarding the pharmacokinetic and pharmacodynamic effects of eptifibatide given at those dose levels, due in part to the overestimation of the pharmacodynamic effects mentioned above—specifically, only 50% of the maximal possible blockade of the glycoprotein IIb/IIIa receptor was achieved with the doses used in IMPACT-II (15). The information gained from PRIDE was used to inform the design of the Phase III Enhanced Suppression of the Platelet IIb/IIIa Receptor with Integrilin Therapy (ESPRIT) study of patients undergoing stent implantation (14,18).
  - The indication of acute MI was not pursued in Phase III testing, perhaps because the IMPACT-AMI trial did not show an improvement with eptifibatide use for the composite in-hospital end point of death, reinfarction, stroke, revascularization, new heart failure, or pulmonary edema, but only for the angiographic and electrocardiographic variables measured (12).
- Although all of the Phase II studies collected information about clinical end points, two studies (IMPACT-AMI and IMPACT-USA)

(12,13) also collected information about effects on electrocardio-graphic or angiographic markers of ischemia, both potential surro-gates for clinical events.

• In terms of evaluating safety, bleeding was the major focus in all of the Phase II studies.

Eptifibatide was developed with the goal of providing a potent anti-platelet agent with a favorable safety profile. Phase I and II studies pro-vided evidence of both adequate inhibition of platelet aggregation and a low risk of bleeding. In Phase I studies, bleeding times were somewhat lengthened with eptifibatide, but they returned to baseline values shortly after stopping the infusion and no clinical bleeding events occurred. In Phase II studies, the incidence of major/severe bleeding and other mea-sures of hemostasis did not differ significantly among the treatment arms. The Phase II studies also determined that eptifibatide could be given safely with other antithrombotic drugs commonly used in patients with heart disease, such as aspirin and heparin. Finally, eptifibatide use revealed no antigenic potential, allowing the possibility of repeated dosing without serious risk of thrombocytopenia or an antibody response. This type of adverse event occurred in about 6% of the patients receiving the only other intravenous antiplatelet agent at that time, abciximab (19). No other safety issues were uncovered during the Phase II studies.

In the Phase II IMPACT trials, sample sizes were too small to show statistically significant effects on clinical outcomes in patients with unsta-ble angina and those undergoing coronary intervention, but there clearly were dose-dependent antithrombotic effects and a trend toward reduced ischemic events, including death, MI, and repeat revascularization. The IMPACT High-Low trial also showed a rapid and rapidly reversible inhib-itory effect of eptifibatide on glycoprotein IIb/IIIa and provided guidelines for dosing regimens in the subsequent Phase III IMPACT-II (17) and PUR-SUIT (16) trials. These studies are discussed further in the next chapter.

CONCLUSION

Phase II clinical development evaluates safety and explores dosing and pharmacodynamic responses to novel therapeutics in a patient population with the disease of interest. The activities of this phase often lead to the critical decision of whether to pursue pivotal Phase III efficacy trials or abandon further development. Sponsors and regulatory agencies increasingly support the use of biomarkers and drug modeling and simulation to improve efficiency and speed the decision-making process. Further efforts to improve efficiency, reduce costs, and improve the generalizability of clinical trial findings through the globalization of Phase II trials have necessarily increased the complexity of even small Phase II studies.

REFERENCES

1. Biomarkers Definitions Working Group. Biomarkers and surrogate endpoints: preferred definitions and conceptual framework. *Clin Pharmacol Ther*. 2001;69(3):89-95.
2. Fleming TR, DeMets DL. Surrogate end points in clinical trials: are we being misled? *Ann Intern Med*. 1996;125(7):605-613.
3. Center for Drug Evaluation and Research, US Food and Drug Administration. Guidance for Industry: End-of-Phase 2A Meetings. 2009. www.fda.gov/downloads/Drugs/GuidanceComplianceRegulatoryInformation/Guidances/UCM079690.pdf Accessed April 17, 2012.
4. Center for Drug Evaluation and Research, US Food and Drug Administration. Draft Guidance for Industry: Adaptive Design Clinical Trials for Drugs and Biologics. 2010. http://www.fda.gov/downloads/Drugs/Guidance ComplianceRegulatoryInformation/Guidances/UCM201790.pdf.
5. International Conference on Harmonisation of Technical Requirements for Registration of Pharmaceuticals for Human Use. E7. Studies in Support of Special Populations: Geriatrics. 1993. http://www.ich.org/fileadmin/Public_Web_Site/ICH_Products/Guidelines/Efficacy/E7/Step4/E7_Guideline.pdf. Accessed April 17, 2012.
6. International Conference on Harmonisation of Technical Requirements for Registration of Pharmaceuticals for Human Use. E11. Clinical Investigation of Medicinal Products in the Pediatric Population. 2000. http://www.ich.org/fileadmin/Public_Web_Site/ICH_Products/Guidelines/Efficacy/E11/Step4/E11_Guideline.pdf. Accessed April 17, 2012.
7. Glickman SW, et al. Ethical and scientific implications of the globalization of clinical research. *N Engl J Med*. 2009;360(8):816-823.
8. Hanson J, et al. Progress in the field of GPIIb/IIIa antagonists. *Curr Med Chem Cardiovasc Hematol Agents*. 2004;2(2):157-167.
9. Scarborough RM. Development of eptifibatide. *Am Heart J*. 1999;138(6 Pt 1):1093-1104.
10. Tcheng JE, et al. Multicenter, randomized, double-blind, placebo-controlled trial of the platelet integrin glycoprotein IIb/IIIa blocker Integrelin in elective coronary intervention. IMPACT Investigators. *Circulation*. 1995;91(8):2151-2157.

11. Harrington RA, et al. Immediate and reversible platelet inhibition after intravenous administration of a peptide glycoprotein IIb/IIIa inhibitor during percutaneous coronary intervention. *Am J Cardiol.* 1995;76(17):1222-1227.

12. Ohman EM, et al. Combined accelerated tissue-plasminogen activator and platelet glycoprotein IIb/IIIa integrin receptor blockade with Integrilin in acute myocardial infarction. Results of a randomized, placebo-controlled, dose-ranging trial. IMPACT-AMI Investigators. *Circulation.* 1997;95(4):846-854.

13. Schulman SP, et al. Effects of integrelin, a platelet glycoprotein IIb/IIIa receptor antagonist, in unstable angina. A randomized multicenter trial. *Circulation.* 1996;94(9):2083-2089.

14. Tcheng JE, et al. Clinical pharmacology of higher dose eptifibatide in percutaneous coronary intervention (the PRIDE study). *Am J Cardiol.* 2001;88 (10):1097-1102.

15. Phillips DR, et al. Effect of Ca2+ on GP IIb-IIIa interactions with integrilin: enhanced GP IIb-IIIa binding and inhibition of platelet aggregation by reductions in the concentration of ionized calcium in plasma anticoagulated with citrate. *Circulation.* 1997;96(5):1488-1494.

16. The PURSUIT Trial Investigators. Inhibition of platelet glycoprotein IIb/IIIa with eptifibatide in patients with acute coronary syndromes. *N Engl J Med.* 1998; 339(7):436-443.

17. Integrilin to Minimise Platelet Aggregation and Coronary Thrombosis-II Investigators. Randomised placebo-controlled trial of effect of eptifibatide on complications of percutaneous coronary intervention: IMPACT-II. *Lancet.* 1997;349(9063):1422-1428.

18. ESPRIT Investigators. Novel dosing regimen of eptifibatide in planned coronary stent implantation (ESPRIT): a randomised, placebo-controlled trial (erratum in Lancet 2001;357(9265):1370). *Lancet.* 2000;356(9247):2037-2044.

19. The EPILOG Investigators. Platelet glycoprotein IIb/IIIa receptor blockade and low-dose heparin during percutaneous coronary revascularization. *N Engl J Med.* 1997;336(24):1689-1696.

CHAPTER EIGHT

Phase III and IV Clinical Trials

Gail E. Hafley, Sergio Leonardi, and Karen S. Pieper

PHASE III TRIALS

Phase III trials are typically undertaken after Phase II studies have identified a potentially safe and effective dose that is considered likely to show an effect on a relevant clinical end point. Typically, regulatory approval in the United States requires two statistically significant, well-controlled clinical trials for the same indication.

Phase III trials usually enroll several hundred to several thousand subjects at multiple study centers. The major objective in Phase III is to show a statistically significant effect on the relevant efficacy measure to facilitate approval of the drug by regulatory agencies, confirming evidence collected in Phase II that a drug is safe and effective for use in the intended indication and population. Secondary objectives can include evaluating safety and dosing for package labeling; its use in subpopulations, wider populations, and with other medications; and effects on secondary end points (1) (Table 8–1).

Phase III trials show efficacy by comparing the new therapy to a control, which can be standard therapy, no therapy, or a placebo. The most frequently used trial design is the superiority trial, which aims to show that the new therapy is better than the comparator. When effective treatments for a condition are already available, however, showing superiority against these treatments can be much more difficult than showing it against a placebo. In some cases, such large numbers of patients would be needed to declare superiority that performing such a trial becomes prohibitive. It may be more reasonable to show that the new therapy is equivalent or

TABLE 8–1
Objectives of a Phase III study
• Confirm the efficacy of the therapy • Monitor adverse events and side effects • Compare effectiveness relative to current therapies • Describe the benefit/risk ratio across different types of patients

noninferior to existing standard therapy with regard to efficacy and safety while also showing other characteristics that make it desirable, for example, fewer side effects, shorter half-life, easier to give, or less expensive. The goal of an equivalence trial is to show that the effects of the new therapy differ by no more than a clinically acceptable amount from those of the comparative therapy, whereas the goal of a noninferiority trial is to show that any difference in effectiveness between the new therapy and the control is not worse by a clinically meaningful amount.

Phase III trials are frequently designed to include specified interim "looks" at the data by an independent committee composed of knowledgeable experts, often referred to as a Data and Safety Monitoring Board (DSMB). This committee assesses the available trial data to determine whether there is sufficient cause for stopping the trial early or modifying trial conduct. Reasons for early stopping include a clear indication that the treatment is superior, a low likelihood of achieving the specified treatment benefit, unacceptable adverse events, and patient accrual that is too slow to complete the study in a timely manner. During an interim look, numerous quantitative methods can be used to evaluate the data for a clear indication that the treatment is superior. The most widely accepted methods used in current clinical trials are frequentist procedures, such as group-sequential boundaries. With these methods, critical values for hypothesis-testing are set for each evaluation of the end point such that the overall Type I error criteria will be satisfied and thus the Type I error rate will be controlled. Clinical trials are also terminated if there is little chance, given the currently available data, that a treatment will be beneficial. Conditional power and predictive power are two methods available for assessing the futility of continuing the trial. Regardless of the methods used to evaluate interim data, interpreting the data and making decisions about early stopping are difficult and often error-prone. Although quantitative methods of evaluation are important, it is critical to have a knowledgeable and experienced DSMB evaluate all aspects of the trial and make decisions based on all information available to them and not on statistical tests alone.

The most widely used treatment-allocation method in a clinical trial is randomization. Randomization is an effective way to reduce selection bias because a patient's treatment assignment is based on chance. A simple randomization assigns treatment to a patient without regard for treatment assignments already made for other patients. This type of randomization can cause undesirable effects in a clinical trial, such as an imbalance in the number of patients in each treatment group or an imbalance among important prognostic factors. Although statistical methods are available to account for imbalances, large differences in important prognostic factors between treatment groups can raise credibility issues.

To prevent these imbalances, blocking is often used in randomization schemes. A block is a number of treatment assignments specified in advance, with the block size being an integer multiple of the number of treatment groups. The order of treatments within a block is randomly permuted, but the number of each treatment is balanced within each block. For example, in a block size of four, one can have the following six blocks: AABB, ABAB, ABBA, BBAA, BABA, and BAAB. A block is picked at random, and that block defines the first set of treatment assignments (Figure 8-1). For this design of a block size of four, the most that the treatment allocations could differ within any one center is by two.

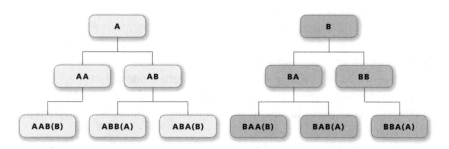

FIGURE 8–1. Illustration of all possible blocks of four for a study of two treatments, A and B. The first treatment assignment is A or B (Row 1). The second assignment is A or B, yielding AA, AB, BA, and BB for all possible treatment assignments to two patients (Row 2). The third assignment yields AAB, ABB, ABA, BAA, BAB, and BBA for all possible treatment assignments to three patients (Row 3). Because there must be two, and only two, of each treatment in each block of four assignments, AA and BB can be followed only by B and A, respectively, and the fourth treatment assignment is fixed.

All blocks do not need to be the same size. As illustrated in Figure 8-1, if investigators can determine the treatments that patients receive (or think they can), then once the first three treatments in a block are given, the assignment to the fourth patient would be known. This could influence the investigator's decision to enroll a particular patient to receive that fourth assignment. To control for this, a random block design may be used. In this case, blocks that are multiples of the number of treatments are developed. For our two-treatment study, these could be block sizes of two, four, six, etc. Treatment allocation within large Phase III trials is often blocked within each center, resulting in a nearly balanced number of patients in each treatment group at each center.

Other types of treatment allocation include dynamic or adaptive allocation methods. Minimization and biased coin are two types of such methods. Minimization tries to balance treatment allocation across important prognostic factors. This method uses the levels of the stratification factors of the patients already in the trial, the treatment of each, and the values of these factors for the next patient in determining the treatment assignment for this next patient. An imbalance score is created for the patient for each treatment assignment, and the treatment with the smallest score is assigned. For the biased coin, a patient is randomly allocated to the treatment arm with fewer patients with a probability $P > 0.5$. In the adaptive biased coin design, the value of P depends on the level of imbalance in the number of patients already allocated to each arm.

When evaluating efficacy outcomes, the principle of *intention to treat* (ITT) is generally applied. According to the ITT principle, the statistical analysis includes patients in the treatment group to which they were assigned through randomization. Thus, patients who die or withdraw before being treated, receive the wrong treatment, or switch from one treatment group to another during the study are still considered, for the main efficacy analyses, to have received the therapy to which they were randomized. This method preserves the assumption of random allocation of therapy. It also reduces potential bias that could result from selecting patients to preferentially receive one treatment or another.

In some trials there may be reasonable cause to eliminate one or more patients from the ITT analysis (e.g., there may be patients randomized who do not meet entry criteria, patients not exposed to study treatment, or patients lost to follow-up.) Analysis of a modified ITT (MITT) population excluding these patients may still be in accordance with ITT principles, provided that the mechanism for excluding patients is not associated with treatment assignment. To avoid concerns about potential inflation of Type I error, it is best to describe

the plan for any MITT analyses in the protocol. A large number of unantici-
pated exclusions from the ITT could raise concerns about the conduct of
a trial.

To acquire a comprehensive safety profile for new therapies, safety
outcomes are typically analyzed according to treatment received and not
randomized treatment. Patients are assessed for routine safety endpoints
from the time they are first exposed to study treatment until a specified
time point after their last exposure to the treatment—e.g., 30 days or 60
days. Serious and unexpected adverse events occurring after the end of
planned follow-up are generally reported to the license holder of the study
treatment and the appropriate regulatory authorities.

The amount of missing data has a substantial effect on the overall quality
of clinical trials (2). The problem can be especially severe with longer trials
and those with incomplete ascertainment of fatal and nonfatal end points. For
this reason, it is usually important to make a clear distinction in the protocol
between nonadherence (i.e., not receiving a randomized intervention) and
nonretention (i.e., not ascertaining the end point of interest). The occurrence
of side effects, inability to tolerate the intervention, toxicity, or need for other
therapies can be valid reasons for nonadherence, but not for nonretention.
Ideally, the only valid reason for nonretention is the withdrawal of consent.
Nonretention rates of >1% could bring into question the study results.

Phase III Studies of Eptifibatide

With the promising results from the Phase II trials of eptifibatide, a Phase
III trial, Integrilin to Minimise Platelet Aggregation and Coronary Thrombosis (IMPACT)-II (3), began enrollment in November 1993. This was a
randomized, double-blinded, placebo-controlled superiority trial in
patients scheduled for elective, urgent, or emergency coronary intervention with a US Food and Drug Administration (FDA)-approved device
(balloon angioplasty, directional coronary atherectomy, rotational atherectomy, or excimer laser ablation). Within a year, 4,010 patients were
enrolled at 82 centers in the United States.

The primary end point was the occurrence within 30 days of death,
myocardial infarction (MI), urgent or emergency repeat coronary intervention, urgent or emergency coronary artery bypass surgery, or placement of
an intracoronary stent in the index vessel because of abrupt closure. The
primary analysis was to be performed by ITT. Several secondary end points
were also prospectively defined (Table 8–2).

TABLE 8-2

Characteristics of two Phase III trials of eptifibatide

	IMPACT-II	PURSUIT
Objectives	Efficacy Safety	Efficacy Safety
Study population	Patients scheduled for elective, urgent, or emergency coronary intervention[a]	Patients with unstable angina or non–Q-wave MI
Sample size	4,010	10,948
Enrollment period	Nov 1993–Nov 1994	Nov 1995–Jan 1997
Primary end point(s)	Clinical composite[b] at 30 days	Death or MI at 30 days
Other end points	Clinical composite[b] at 24 hours and 6 months, clinical composite[b] as determined by investigator, abrupt closure on angiogram, major bleeding, blood transfusion, stroke	Death or MI at 96 hours, 7 days, and 6 months
Study design	Randomized Multicenter Double-blind	Randomized Multicenter (worldwide) Double-blind
Treatment arms	Eptifibatide bolus and 0.5-μg/kg/min infusion Eptifibatide bolus and 0.75-μg/kg/min infusion Placebo bolus and infusion	Eptifibatide bolus and 2.0-μg/kg/min infusion Eptifibatide bolus and 1.3-μg/kg/min infusion Placebo bolus and infusion

[a]Balloon angioplasty, directional coronary atherectomy, high-speed rotational atherectomy, or excimer laser ablation.
[b]All-cause mortality, myocardial infarction (MI), urgent or emergency repeat coronary intervention, urgent or emergency coronary artery bypass surgery, or index placement of an intracoronary stent for abrupt closure.

Patients were randomly assigned to one of three treatment arms: an eptifibatide bolus with a 0.5-μg/kg/min infusion (low dose), an eptifibatide bolus with a 0.75-μg/kg/min infusion (high dose), and a placebo bolus with placebo infusion (placebo). The trial was designed to detect a 33% reduction in the primary end point in either or both eptifibatide treatment arms compared with placebo, with 80% power and $\alpha = 0.05$. To adjust for multiple tests, a significance level of <0.035 was used for each comparison to ensure that the Type I error rate for both comparisons was <0.05. The original planned sample size was 3,500 patients. An O'Brien–Fleming group-sequential design was used to define stopping rules for the three interim efficacy analyses. At the conclusion of the third interim analysis, the DSMB recommended that the sample size be increased to 4,000 patients because of a lower-than-expected event rate in the placebo arm.

Randomization occurred before the decision to perform a coronary intervention was made. This resulted in 3.5% of patients not receiving study drug and 3.1% not undergoing coronary intervention. The investigators thought that in addition to the ITT analysis, it was important to evaluate the treatment benefit in patients who actually received the study drug. Thus, the protocol was amended to allow comparison of the ITT groups, but including only treated patients.

The results of the protocol-specified ITT analysis (all randomized patients) showed nonsignificant reductions in the primary composite end point of 21% for the low-dose group ($P = 0.063$) and 14% for the high-dose group ($P = 0.22$) compared with placebo. After excluding the 139 patients who did not receive treatment, there was a significant 22% reduction ($P = 0.035$) in the primary end point in the low-dose group compared with placebo, whereas results in the high-dose group remained unchanged at a 14% reduction ($P = 0.178$). Incidence of the composite end point at 24 hours was significantly reduced in both treatment arms compared with placebo. At 6 months, the results were similar to those obtained at 30 days. The study also showed an excellent safety profile for eptifibatide—bleeding and other adverse event rates were similar across all three treatment groups.

After the completion of IMPACT-II, new findings revealed that its dosing regimens were at the low end of the dose–response curve and that the significant early benefits were probably attributable to the bolus dose, suggesting that a higher dose may lead to greater benefit. The efficacy of an increased dose was tested in the Platelet glycoprotein IIb/IIIa in Unstable angina: Receptor Suppression Using Integrilin Therapy (PURSUIT) trial (4), a double-blinded, placebo-controlled superiority study of eptifibatide that enrolled 10,948 patients with unstable angina or non–Q-wave

MI at 700 centers in 28 countries. The primary end point of the study was the occurrence within 30 days of the composite end point of death or MI as adjudicated by a clinical events committee. Several secondary end points were also prospectively defined (Table 8–2).

Patients who had ischemic chest pain within the previous 24 hours and had either electrocardiographic changes indicative of ischemia or an elevated creatine kinase-MB level were randomized to receive one of three treatments: an eptifibatide bolus with a 2.0-μg/kg/min infusion (high dose), an eptifibatide bolus with a 1.3-μg/kg/min infusion (low dose), or a placebo bolus and infusion (placebo). The protocol specified that the low-dose arm would be dropped if the DSMB's review of safety data found the higher dose to be acceptable. After 3,218 patients had been randomized, the DSMB did recommend that the lower dose be dropped. From then on, patients were randomized to receive either the high dose or placebo; the primary analysis was based on these two treatment arms alone. An O'Brien–Fleming type approach was used to define stopping boundaries for four interim looks by the DSMB.

There was a significant reduction in the primary end point of death or MI at 30 days (14.2% versus 15.7%; $P = 0.042$). The reduction in events occurred within 96 hours of treatment and continued throughout the 30 days. The effect of eptifibatide varied among regions, with the greatest benefit occurring in the United States and no effect seen in Eastern Europe or Latin America. Bleeding and transfusion of red blood cells were more frequent among patients treated with eptifibatide, although in most cases the bleeding was mild.

At the conclusion of PURSUIT, the FDA approved eptifibatide therapy for use in patients with non–ST-segment elevation MI or unstable angina (5).

PHASE IV TRIALS

After Phase III trials have been completed and the treatment of interest has been favorably reviewed by the FDA and/or by regulatory bodies for countries outside the United States, additional studies may be performed. These usually fall under the category of Phase IV studies. They also may be considered to be part of a postapproval surveillance effort. Postapproval (also termed postmarketing) surveillance includes several nonstudy activities, many of which are based on spontaneous reporting (6).

Phase IV studies are often done for drugs that are already approved by the FDA and are being prescribed or given to patients. These studies provide

TABLE 8–3

Objectives of a Phase IV study

• Evaluate risks, side effects, and benefits over longer periods
• Further describe the drug's mechanism of action
• Studies the optimal use of the treatment

additional information about the efficacy, risks, methods of use, and optimal use of a treatment (Table 8–3).

A Phase IV study can occur for a variety of reasons. The FDA may approve the new treatment and require that the manufacturer provide additional long-term surveillance. This surveillance will supplement the data from the Phase III studies with information about efficacy and safety over longer periods. A Phase IV trial can be part of a defined risk evaluation mitigation strategy (REMS), in which case the sample size, expected start and completion dates, and evidence of compliance would need to be included in REMS documentation (7). A Phase IV study may evaluate the efficacy or safety of the treatment in populations not studied in the Phase I–III trials, such as very elderly persons, children, women of childbearing age, or patients with comorbid conditions. It may be used to evaluate interactions with medications that the typical patient may also be taking.

If the purpose of the Phase IV study is to evaluate dosing or to compare a treatment with other standard treatments, then the study design should be similar to that of a Phase III study, with randomization of therapy assignment and blinding both being important factors. If the purpose is surveillance, then the study can be uncontrolled or observational. The follow-up period for surveillance studies can be very long, with thousands of patients being followed.

Phase IV Studies of Eptifibatide

Two Phase IV studies were conducted to study eptifibatide. As discussed, the IMPACT-II trial had shown a reduction in the 30-day composite end point with the use of eptifibatide, but this difference was not dramatic (9.2% versus 11.4% with placebo; $P = 0.063$ in ITT analysis and 9.1% versus 14.6%; $P = 0.035$ in the ITT-treated analysis) (3). The PURSUIT study enrolled a wider range of patients with acute coronary syndromes and showed a similar level of statistical significance for the reduction in the incidence of death or MI at 30 days ($P = 0.042$) (4). In the same year that PURSUIT was published (1998), the Evaluation of Platelet IIb/IIIa Inhibitor for STENTing (EPISTENT) superiority trial showed a highly statistically significant reduction in the incidence of death, MI, or target-vessel revascularization at 30 days in patients undergoing coronary stent implantation who received abciximab (another glycoprotein IIb/IIIa inhibitor) versus placebo ($P < 0.001$) (8).

In 1999, the first patient was enrolled in the Phase IV Enhanced Suppression of the Platelet IIb/IIIa Receptor with Integrilin Therapy (ESPRIT) trial (9). Further studies and pharmacodynamic modeling of eptifibatide had suggested that better blockade of the glycoprotein IIb/IIIa receptor than that seen in IMPACT-II could be obtained using a bolus dose of 180 μg/kg followed by a 2.0-μg/kg/min infusion for 18–24 hours, with a second bolus of 180 μg/kg to follow 10 minutes after the first (10,11). The ESPRIT superiority trial tested the use of this dosing regimen of eptifibatide versus placebo in patients undergoing planned stent implantation.

In some circles, this trial was controversial. Both the IMPACT-II secondary analyses and the PURSUIT main results showed that eptifibatide was superior to placebo for the clinical outcomes tested ($P = 0.035$ and 0.042, respectively). Given these results, the ethics of exposing patients to a placebo were questioned. The leaders of the trial countered that ESPRIT was exploring the treatment of patients during a new era of medicine and that patients would receive different treatments than in the previous studies: newer stents, low-dose heparin, and concomitant treatment with thienopyridines (9).

Unlike IMPACT-II, patients in ESPRIT were randomized in the catheterization laboratory only after angiography confirmed that they would proceed to stenting, thus greatly diminishing the risk that some randomized patients would receive no treatment and/or no procedure. The final results of the composite end point of death, MI, urgent target vessel revascularization, or thrombotic bailout with glycoprotein IIb/IIIa inhibition within 48 hours of randomization were 6.6% for eptifibatide versus 10.5% for placebo ($P = 0.0015$) (9). Although these results helped boost confidence in the use of eptifibatide in the catheterization laboratory, there was still doubt about the utility of starting the drug in the emergency room.

In May 2004, the first patient was enrolled in the EARLY glycoprotein IIb/IIIa inhibition in non–ST-segment elevation Acute Coronary Syndrome (EARLY-ACS) trial (12). This trial was designed to test whether the strategy of early use of a glycoprotein IIb/IIIa inhibitor would be superior to a delayed strategy, in which the decision to use the drug occurred at the time of percutaneous coronary intervention (PCI). Patients who were expected to undergo PCI no sooner than the next calendar day after randomization were randomized within 8 hours of presentation to receive routine early use of eptifibatide or provisional eptifibatide. Those involved in the study were blinded to treatment assignment. At randomization, patients received either an eptifibatide or placebo bolus, followed by an infusion as specified in the ESPRIT trial. After cardiac catheterization but before PCI, the attending physician could request eptifibatide. At that time, patients randomized to the early eptifibatide arm received a bolus dose of placebo, and those randomized to delayed treatment received a bolus of eptifibatide. The randomized infusion was stopped in both arms, and an open-label infusion of eptifibatide was started and continued for 18–24 hours. The two groups did not differ significantly in the primary outcome of death, MI, recurrent ischemia requiring urgent revascularization, or thrombotic bailout with glycoprotein IIb/IIIa inhibition at 96 hours ($P = 0.23$) (12).

A final example of a Phase IV-like study is the Can Rapid Risk Stratification of Unstable Angina Patients Suppress Adverse Outcomes with Early Implementation of the ACC/AHA Guidelines? (CRUSADE) registry (13). CRUSADE was designed as a quality improvement and educational initiative for emergency departments and cardiologists seeing high-risk patients with non–ST-segment elevation acute coronary syndromes. Participating centers received feedback about their use of treatments recommended by the American College of Cardiology/American Heart Association guidelines compared with national norms, and educational programs and scientific publications provided additional reinforcement of the appropriate use of these treatments. This registry provided a valuable tool to improve patient care. One example is the study of antithrombotic dosing in the CRUSADE population. Alexander et al. found that the patients who received excess dosing also had a higher rate of major bleeding (14). Given that no study can ethically be performed to examine under- or overdosing of an accepted drug, this information is valuable in helping guide dosing decisions for antithrombotic therapies.

On January 1, 2007, CRUSADE merged with the National Registry for Myocardial Infarction (NRMI) to become the Acute Coronary Treatment and Intervention Outcomes Network (ACTION®) of the National Cardiovascular Data Registry (NCDR), which was run at the time by the American College of Cardiology (15). This combined dataset was then merged in June 2008 with the Get With The Guidelines® program of the American Heart Association (16).

CONCLUSION

Phase III trials are based on the accumulated information from Phase I and II clinical trials as well as studies of similar compounds. They provide information about the benefit–risk profile of the treatment and advance understanding of the patient response to treatment, to be the basis for governmental approval for marketing. Phase IV studies continue to provide information about the safety of the treatment, other possible uses of the treatment, and optimization of dose.

REFERENCES

1. US Food and Drug Administration. Development & Approval Process (Drugs). 2009. http://www.fda.gov/drugs/developmentapprovalprocess/default .htm. Accessed April 23, 2012.
2. Fleming TR. Addressing missing data in clinical trials. *Ann Intern Med.* 2011;154(2):113-117.
3. Integrilin to Minimise Platelet Aggregation and Coronary Thrombosis-II Investigators. Randomised placebo-controlled trial of effect of eptifibatide on complications of percutaneous coronary intervention: IMPACT-II. *Lancet.* 1997;349(9063):1422-1428.
4. The PURSUIT Trial Investigators. Inhibition of platelet glycoprotein IIb/IIIa with eptifibatide in patients with acute coronary syndromes. *N Engl J Med.* 1998;339(7):436-443.
5. US Food and Drug Administration. Drug Approval Package: Integrilin (eptifibatide) injection. 1998. http://www.accessdata.fda.gov/drugsatfda_docs/ nda/ 98/20718_Integrilin.cfm. Accessed April 10, 2012.
6. US Food and Drug Administration. Guidance, Compliance, & Regulatory Information. 2012. http://www.fda.gov/Drugs/GuidanceComplianceRegula toryInformation/default.htm. Accessed April 23, 2012.
7. Center for Drug Evaluation and Research, US Food and Drug Administration. Surveillance – Postmarketing Surveillance Programs. 2009. http:// www.fda.gov/Drugs/GuidanceComplianceRegulatoryInformation/Surveil lance/ucm090385.htm. Accessed April 23, 2012.
8. EPISTENT Investigators. Randomised placebo-controlled and balloon-angioplasty-controlled trial to assess safety of coronary stenting with use of platelet glycoprotein-IIb/IIIa blockade. *Lancet.* 1998;352(9122):87-92.
9. ESPRIT Investigators. Novel dosing regimen of eptifibatide in planned coronary stent implantation (ESPRIT): a randomised, placebo-controlled trial (erratum in Lancet. 2001;357(9265):1370). *Lancet.* 2000;356(9247):2037-2044.

10. Tcheng JE, et al. Clinical pharmacology of higher dose eptifibatide in percutaneous coronary intervention (the PRIDE study). *Am J Cardiol.* 2001;88 (10):1097-1102.

11. Gilchrist IC, et al. Pharmacodynamics and pharmacokinetics of higher-dose, double-bolus eptifibatide in percutaneous coronary intervention. *Circulation.* 2001;104(4):406-411.

12. Giugliano RP, et al. Early versus delayed, provisional eptifibatide in acute coronary syndromes. *N Engl J Med.* 2009;360(21):2176-2190.

13. Hoekstra JW, et al. Improving the care of patients with non-ST-elevation acute coronary syndromes in the emergency department: the CRUSADE initiative. *Acad Emerg Med.* 2002;9(11):1146-1155.

14. Alexander KP, et al. Excess dosing of antiplatelet and antithrombin agents in the treatment of non-ST-segment elevation acute coronary syndromes. *JAMA.* 2005;294(24):3108-3116.

15. National Cardiovascular Disease Registry. NCDR® ACTION Registry®-GWTG™ Home Page. http://www.ncdr.com/WebNCDR/Action/default.aspx. Accessed April 23, 2012.

16. Peterson ED, et al. A call to ACTION (Acute Coronary Treatment and Intervention Outcomes Network): a national effort to promote timely clinical feedback and support continuous quality improvement for acute myocardial infarction. *Circ Cardiovasc Qual Outcomes.* 2009;2(5):491-499.

CHAPTER NINE

Challenges of Clinical Trials in Pediatrics

Kevin N. Turner and P. Brian Smith

HOUSTON, WE HAVE A PROBLEM

*J*anna was a 3-month-old baby who had survived neonatal cardiac surgery with a good prognosis. Not unlike other young children, Janna suffered from gastroesophageal reflux and was receiving cisapride. One morning, she was noted to be fussy while in her swing chair and, within 10 minutes, became unresponsive.

Cisapride was a medication approved by the US Food and Drug Administration (FDA) in 1993 for nighttime heartburn in adults. It was never shown to be effective or safe in children under the age of 16 and therefore had no FDA approval for use in this population (1,2). However, cisapride quickly found a market treating a common neonatal problem, gastroesophageal reflux (GER). There was a flavored syrup formulation that was labeled for use in geriatrics, but 90% of its sales were for use in pediatric patients (3). Hospitalized preterm infants also receive medications for symptoms thought to be associated with GER, including apnea, bradycardia, coughing, choking, and cyanosis (4,5). By 1998, more than 19% of infants in neonatal intensive care units (NICUs) in the United States were receiving cisapride (4).

In 1995, a case report had been published of a particular arrhythmia, prolonged QT interval, in a 64-year-old patient taking high-dose cisapride (6). QT prolongation, although not independently dangerous, can lead to the fatal arrhythmia torsades de pointes, especially during episodes of bradycardia. Additionally, erythromycin, commonly used in infants, was found to carry a particularly high risk of fatal arrhythmia when coadministered with cisapride, both by inhibiting its metabolism and by exaggerating ion channel disturbances that cause QT changes (4). By 2000, after 80 deaths and 341 serious adverse events had been reported, mostly in children, cisapride was pulled from general use in the US market (4,6,7).

Cisapride is just one example of many therapeutics often used in children despite a paucity of safety, dosing, and efficacy data. Trimethoprim/sulfamethoxazole, an antibiotic that was deemed safe to use in children, is another. In the 1950s, physicians recognized that infants who received the antibiotic prophylactically had a much higher incidence of kernicterus, a permanent neurological complication of hyperbilirubinemia. Transient hyperbilirubinemia is present in every newborn, and kernicterus is a complication observed almost exclusively in this population. Therefore, kernicterus had not previously been described during the use of trimethoprim/sulfamethoxazole in adults. After this association was noted, studies in animals found that trimethoprim/sulfamethoxazole displaced bilirubin from albumin, increasing the risk of kernicterus in newborns (8).

In the late 1990s, premature infants often received prophylactic steroids to prevent chronic lung disease. Although steroids never received FDA approval for this indication, several randomized trials did show short-term benefits (9,10). When long-term neurodevelopment was examined, however, steroids were associated with a significant increase in the risk of cerebral palsy (11,12).

In 1963, Dr. Harry Shirkey coined the term "therapeutic orphans" to describe children, owing to the lack of active research dedicated to defining the optimal dosing, safety, and efficacy of therapeutics in this population (13). Historically, up to 75% of drugs have had insufficient labeling for pediatric safety, efficacy, and dosing. This percentage is even higher for drugs used in infants. Infants are at particular risk for inaccurate dosing, and an estimated 90% of patients in NICUs receive at least one medication "off-label" (14). Moreover, medication use in this population is on the rise; currently NICU patients receive a median of eight drugs (15).

CHILDREN ARE NOT LITTLE ADULTS

It is 8:15 a.m., and Dr. Roberts has seen her first two patients of the morning, with dozens to follow, not uncommon in January. Sarah is a 9-month-old ex-premature infant who weighed <500 g at birth and who now has acute otitis media. Ryan is an obese 17-year-old, weighing 130 kg, who has bacterial sinusitis. Dr. Roberts plans to treat both patients with high-dose amoxicillin to cover for resistant Streptococcus pneumoniae. She steps back *into her office to use her calculator to determine the correct dosing for each.*

Before 1962, there were no requirements for human testing of new pharmaceuticals. The Kefauver–Harris Amendment (Table 9–1) was partly inspired by the case of thalidomide, a drug widely used to treat morning sickness in pregnant women in the early 1960s (15,16). After its release,

TABLE 9–1
Time line of efforts to improve pediatric drug safety (15,16)

Year	Title	Description
1906	Pure Food and Drugs Act	Inception of drug regulation
1938	Federal Food, Drug, and Cosmetic Act	Required safety documentation and toxicity studies
1962	Kefauver–Harris Amendment	Established three phases of drug trials and required preclinical testing
1979	Pediatric information requirements	Established a section for pediatric drug labels
1994	Pediatric drug labeling	Required sponsors to examine current evidence for sufficiency of pediatric labeling. Implemented voluntary plan to support pediatric use
1997	Food and Drug Administration Modernization Act (FDAMA)	Provided 6-month extension of patent protection to sponsors that conduct studies in children
1998	Pediatric Rule	FDA required pediatric trials of new drugs if they had potential for use in children
2002	Pediatric Rule overturned	Federal District Court ruled that FDA overstepped its authority
2002	Best Pharmaceuticals For Children Act (BPCA)	Extended FDAMA provisions, authorized National Institutes of Health (NIH) collaboration with FDA to fund pediatric studies for off-label medications
2003	Pediatric Research Equity Act (PREA)	Codified the Pediatric Rule
2007	FDA Amendments Act (FDAAA)	Reauthorized BPCA and PREA provisions
2010	NIH Pediatric Trials Network (PTN)	NIH established a network for developing and conducting therapeutic and device trials in children

thalidomide was found to be teratogenic, resulting in many significant birth defects. The Amendment codified the current three-phase process of investigating new drugs, wherein safety and pharmacokinetic trials are performed in the first phase, efficacy and dosing ranges are established during the second phase, and comparative experimental clinical trials with further refinement on efficacy and dosing are explored during the third phase. Historically, the FDA did not request pediatric studies until Phase III trials had been completed in adults. Although deemed ethically appropriate to conclude adult clinical trials before exposing children to new therapeutics, data were often extrapolated from adults to estimate the pharmacokinetics, safety, and efficacy of new drugs in children (17).

As children develop, however, their continuous changes in physiology affect drug absorption, distribution, metabolism, and excretion. These changes are most evident in premature infants (Table 9–2). As an example, micafungin was found to require up to a fivefold increase in dosing (on a

---

TABLE 9–2

Developmental changes in physiology—effects of pediatric drug disposition

Pharmacokinetic profiles	Difference in infants compared with adults
Absorption: erratic and unpredictable	• GI function: Reduced gastric acid secretion, prolonged gastric emptying, increased intestinal absorptive surface area, increased intestinal transit time, decreased bile acid pool, and irregular peristalsis • Blood flow: Inconsistent blood flow to sites of medication administration (muscle, fat) • Skin: Thinner skin stratum and increased hydration affecting permeability
Drug distribution: a changing continuum	• Body: Higher percentage of total body water, lower percentage of body fat • Plasma protein: Lower level of plasma proteins and thus fewer drug–protein binding sites • CNS: Immature blood–brain barrier causing increased CNS effects
Metabolism and excretion: immature organs	• Liver: Drug-metabolizing enzymes mature to adult levels at varying ages • Renal: Lower glomerular filtration rates, reduced renal blood flow, reduced tubular function

CNS, central nervous system, GI gastrointestinal.

per-kg basis) in premature infants compared with adults (18–20). Age and its effect on organ maturation are of particular importance in dosing, although weight- or body surface area (BSA)-based dosing alone is often entertained. This difficulty is augmented for pediatricians, whose patients can vary in weight by 300-fold.

Drug absorption in children can differ markedly from that in adults, producing unpredictable drug concentrations after oral dosing. Many physiological factors unique to young patients affect drug bioavailability. Gastric pH is elevated in infants because of both the reduced total volume of gastric secretions and reduced parietal cell function. This results in increased absorption of orally administered acid-labile drugs and decreased absorption of drugs that are weak acids (21–23). Gastric emptying time decreases rapidly during the first week of life, whereas intestinal transit time matures rapidly during early infancy (24). Splanchnic blood flow matures during the first 3 weeks of life. These factors contribute to rapidly changing absorption rates during the first several weeks after birth, and by 4 months of age, these processes approach adult levels (14,17,23,25). Gastrointestinal physiology is equivalent to that in adults by age 10–12 years, although erratic eating habits in the adolescent can continue to contribute to skewed bioavailability (23,26,27).

Infants have proportionately less muscle mass and reduced muscle blood flow compared with adults, leading to slowed absorption of intramuscularly administered drugs (17,23,26). Topically applied drugs are affected by differences in skin permeability between adults and infants. Neonatal skin has a thinner stratum, causing increased permeability. The ratio of infants' BSA to their weight is increased relative to older patients, leading to greater topical absorption (23,27). Infants have a sparse amount of body fat and increased extracellular and total body water compared with older children, affecting the distribution of lipid- and water-soluble drugs. They also have reduced protein binding of drugs, resulting in higher levels of unbound active medication and possible toxicity despite having normal serum concentrations (23,28).

Reduced renal blood flow, lower glomerular filtration rates, and functionally immature renal tubules delay renal excretion of drugs. The liver matures markedly during the first few years of life. The cytochrome P (CYP) 450 metabolic pathway is fully functional by age 3 years (17,27). Conjugation to bile salts, a liver function that aids gastrointestinal and renal excretion, matures at age 3–4 years (14,17,23).

All of these factors contribute to inaccuracies in dosing/safety when extrapolating adult information to children.

THE ETHICS OF CLINICAL RESEARCH
IN CHILDREN

Janice is an 8-year-old, prepubescent healthy girl. Her best friend suffers from precocious puberty, which is embarrassing to her, and she regularly visits an endocrinologist. Janice is fascinated by biology and joins her friend on a clinic visit. There she notices a flyer recruiting healthy volunteers for a study to help characterize puberty onset. Her scientific interest piqued, and trying to be supportive of her friend's plight, she excitedly volunteers. The study requires 12 blood samples over a 6-week period.

Ethical principles protecting human subjects (respect for persons, beneficence, and justice) apply to both adult and pediatric subjects. Children require additional considerations, however, as they represent a particularly vulnerable population of study subjects (29).

Paramount to human clinical trials is willing participation. Because minors cannot legally give consent to participate (although clearly they should be involved in the consent process), the FDA requires consent from a minor's parent or legal representative. Studies with higher levels of risk require the consent of both parents, if present. The consent process in children is similar to that in adult subjects, wherein clear language and written documentation are provided. The distinction lies in the requirement for children to also provide assent to the study when developmentally appropriate. Federal regulations stipulate that assent is "a child's affirmative agreement to participate in research," and "mere failure to object should not, absent affirmative agreement, be construed as assent" (29).

Institutional review boards (IRBs) are responsible for ensuring that adequate provisions have been made for soliciting the assent of children. Although no federal stipulation exists, the American Association of Pediatrics suggests that a child is deemed cognitively able to give assent only at the intellectual age of 7 or beyond. Additionally, if the IRB has determined that assent by the child is required for a particular study, the child's dissent prevails, even over the parents' permission. The initial assent is not sufficient, however, and the IRB has the ethical responsibility to ensure ongoing evaluation to confirm the child's continued assent. At any point in the study, the parent or child can revoke permission, and the study team and IRB must be continually watchful for any reluctance on the part of either party (29). Despite these efforts, child subjects often report that the pain of blood sampling is much worse than they imagined during the assent process. In one study of healthy volunteers, children as old as 9 years confessed that they were reluctant to withdraw their assent, believing it would upset the doctor and their parents (30).

> *Janice receives praise from her family about her actions in support of her friend and her scientific interest. Silently, by the third lab draw, she is terrified of returning to the clinic. She develops a fear of needles, hates the smell of the latex tourniquet, and quickly comes to despise the kind nurse who repeatedly offers her the same sticker after each visit. In her 8 years, she has not yet developed the poise to gracefully terminate her participation. She quietly, begrudgingly, dutifully completes her part in the study. Years later, she has repeatedly "forgotten" to schedule her own annual health maintenance exams with her internist, secretly fearing he may want routine labs.*

Most first-in-man studies in adults are done in healthy subjects. Specific rules govern the inclusion of healthy children in medical research, however. The US Department of Health and Human Services, under the Children's Health Act of 2000, regulates research in children. Section 45 CFR Part 46, Subpart D, Additional Protections for Children Involved as Subjects in Research (31), defines four categories of research in which children are allowed to participate (Table 9–3). Categories 2 and 3 involve

TABLE 9–3

Categories of research determined by institutional review boards (31)

Category	Description
1	No greater-than-minimal risk
2	Greater-than-minimal risk but presents the prospect of direct benefit to the individual subject
3	Greater-than-minimal risk, with no prospect of direct benefit to the individual subject, but will likely result in generalizable knowledge about the subject's disorder
4	Does not meet the above criteria, but likely will provide further understanding, prevention, or alleviation of serious health problems of children

subjects who have the disease that the study aims to treat. Only when a study poses no greater-than-minimal risk (Category 1) may an investigator enroll healthy pediatric subjects. Individual IRBs are required to determine in what category the research belongs. IRBs vary in their determination of no greater-than-minimal risk; 18% of IRB chairs consider a single blood draw to exceed minimal risk (32). This all but eliminates healthy controls from pediatric trials and creates a paradox wherein affected "controls" are defining norms, a suboptimal scientific standard not commonly faced in adult trials (29,32).

Category 4 was designed to allow for healthy pediatric controls if the research was deemed to be of profound impact to global childhood health and welfare. Although local IRBs assign the category, they are authorized to approve research only in Categories 1–3. Once an IRB determines that a study falls into Category 4, the organization refers the study to the FDA for its approval. From inception of the Act in 2002 through 2008, only nine Category 4 research proposals had been referred to the FDA for approval (32).

SPECIFIC HURDLES IN PEDIATRIC RESEARCH

Table 9–4 presents a summary of the challenges inherent in pediatric clinical research, which fall into the broad categories of lack of evidence, lack of support, physiological impediments, and need for long-term evaluation. To give just one example, pharmacokinetic studies require multiple, timed blood draws, and exposure to the therapy under study. Aside from the psychological burden this poses on willing child participants, there are also physical limits encountered. Vascular access is often difficult to obtain, and children have less circulating blood volume than do adults. Traditional adult pharmacokinetic trials use 10–15 blood samples per subject, each often >3 mL, and pharmacokinetics are defined for each subject and generalized for a population. In a preterm infant who weighs 500 g, who will have a total blood volume of less than three tablespoons, this sampling rate and blood loss are unacceptable.

Approaches in children often rely on sparse (two to three samples per patient) and low-volume (<100 μL) sampling, leading to a higher likelihood of parental consent. This change in sampling frequency allows experimental samples to be collected along with routine blood draws used in standard care of the patient, thus limiting access via central lines and

TABLE 9–4

Major hurdles to pediatric research and proposed solutions

Hurdles	Proposed solutions
Funding	• Legislation: BPCA, FDAAA, PREA
Adult data extrapolated to children, erroneously considered accurate	• More awareness needed regarding this potential for error • Increased awareness will cause increased demand for evidence-based data derived from children
Small circulating blood volume and difficult access in children	• Pooled population pharmacokinetic studies • Dried blood spot and scavenged sampling • Improved sensitivity of sampling assays
Unique end points for toxicities in children, neurodevelopmental impairment	• Funding for long-term follow-up evaluations of clinical trial subjects

BPCA, Best Pharmaceuticals for Children Act; FDAA, Food and Drug Administration Amendment Act; PREA, Pediatric Research Equity Act.

peripheral punctures. Also, safety monitoring of the therapeutic can overlap routine safety monitoring of an ill patient. Use of scavenged samples, samples drawn as standard care but leftover from laboratory use, also can increase the number of samples collected per subject and likelihood of parental consent (33). These samples are then pooled, and the pharmacokinetics of the drug are determined using a population pharmacokinetic analysis.

Population pharmacokinetics were initially developed to ascertain the pharmacokinetics of certain drugs in unique populations that differed from the initial, usually healthy adult subjects described. Population pharmacokinetics use data collected from multiple subjects within one population, statistically relating them via a nonlinear, mixed-effects model to generate estimated mean and median pharmacokinetics. This process can reveal what factors, possibly unrecognized previously, are contributing to this variability, though this is helpful in describing only the population studied. Population pharmacokinetic analysis has a role in pediatric drug research, given its implicit need for sparse sampling and its ability to generate a curve describing pharmacokinetics in different subpopulations of neonates and infants (34). Another new technology in pharmacokinetic analysis is emerging: dried blood spots (DBS). This method can use as little as 15 μL of whole blood, further reducing the volume of blood needed from each patient (33,35).

Both short-term and long-term risks and toxicology are major concerns in children, and these must be followed to properly describe drug safety. Often, the potential risks to children are unclear when translating a drug that has been carefully described in adults. Aspects of inconvenience, pain, fear, and separation from parents and friends deserve unique consideration. Novel toxicity end points, such as effects on organ development and function and on growth and neurodevelopment, must be monitored. Long-term effects on immune, cognitive, skeletal, and behavioral development require large epidemiological studies and are paramount to safety assessment (26,29).

THE FDA CAN HELP

Baby Boy Johnson is a premature, 2-week-old infant who has begun showing signs of overwhelming infection, although his blood cultures have remained negative for bacteria. His physicians suspect an invasive fungal infection, and they have had success using fluconazole in the past. While deciding on the dose, however, they realize that previous studies have suggested doses for infants in this age range that vary by fourfold. Additionally, fluconazole has received FDA approval only to treat children older than 6 months who have mouth infections. There seems to be no consensus on the correct dose for this child, and yet the physicians know that if this infection is not treated promptly and accurately, their patient may die.

Initial attempts by the FDA to encourage labeling information for children were voluntary and had little effect (16). Between 1991 and 1997, sponsors vowed to complete 71 pediatric studies, but finished only 11 (16). This changed in 1997 with the FDA Modernization Act (FDAMA), which provided financial incentives to pharmaceutical companies: manufacturers would be allowed to extend their exclusive patent protection on drugs by 6 months if they conducted studies of their drug in children. These studies were outlined by the FDA in a written request to the manufacturer. The extended patent was not contingent on ultimate approval of pediatric use.

This legislation has been successful in generating pediatric-specific labeling changes. The provision was renewed in the Best Pharmaceuticals for Children Act (BPCA) of 2002 and again in the FDA Administration Act of 2007 (FDAAA) (36). Combined, these programs have generated 399 pediatric studies and have resulted in labeling changes in 438 drugs for use in children as of April 2012 (37,38).

Although this exclusivity program was voluntary, the Pediatric Rule, enacted in 1998, required manufacturers of all new drugs seeking FDA approval to perform pediatric clinical trials for therapeutics that have the potential to be used in children. Although the Pediatric Rule was eventually overturned, the Pediatric Research Equity Act (PREA) was passed in 2003 and renewed in 2007. This Act required that all new therapeutics submitted for FDA approval have assessed the therapy for use in children unless granted a waiver for unlikely use in children. PREA also required that information generated during pediatric trials be included in the labeling.

The PREA has been successful in generating new understanding of drug disposition in children, but it only captures studies of on-patent drugs. Under the BPCA, Congress gave the FDA a mechanism to consider off-patent medications through a collaborative effort with the National Institutes of Health (NIH) (13–17,37,39).

WHAT WE ARE DOING RIGHT

The Children's Oncology Group (COG) was established in 1955 by the National Cancer Institute. At that time, the cure rate for pediatric cancer was <10%. Today, 90% of pediatric cancers diagnosed in this country are treated at a COG facility. COG offers an extensive handbook to new patients and their families, including describing overarching themes in cancer treatment, such as staging and chemotherapy, and providing substantial information about clinical trials. In clear terms and with diagrams, the handbook describes clinical trials, randomization, the importance of trials, and consent. This initial priming results in 60% of all pediatric cancer patients volunteering to be involved in clinical trials (up to 90% among children with acute lymphoblastic leukemia), compared with about 3% of adult cancer patients (40). Overall, children with cancer can now expect a 5-year survival rate of 83% (41). These efforts are unmatched in adults.

REFERENCES

1. Wysowski DK, Corken A, Gallo-Torres H, Talarico L, Rodriguez EM. Post-marketing reports of QT prolongation and ventricular arrhythmia in association with cisapride and Food and Drug Administration regulatory actions. *Am J Gastroenterol.* 2001;96(6):1698-1703.

2. *Propulsid (Cisapride) Prescribing Information.* Titusville, NJ: Janssen Pharmaceutica; 2006.

3. Harris G, Koli E. Lucrative Drug, Danger Signals and the F.D.A. *The New York Times.* 2005. http://www.nytimes.com/2005/06/10/business/10drug.html. Accessed April 24, 2012.

4. Ward RM, Lemons JA, Molteni RA. Cisapride: a survey of the frequency of use and adverse events in premature newborns. *Pediatrics.* 1999;103(2): 469-472.

5. Malcolm WF, et al. Use of medications for gastroesophageal reflux at discharge among extremely low birth weight infants. *Pediatrics.* 2008;121(1):22-27.

6. Lewin MB, Bryant RM, Fenrich AL, Grifka RG. Cisapride-induced long QT interval. *J Pediatr.* 1996;128(2):279-281.

7. Henney JE. From the Food and Drug Administration. *JAMA.* 2000;283(21): 2779.

8. Ahlfors CE. Bilirubin-albumin binding and free bilirubin. *J Perinatol.* 2001;21 (suppl) 1:S40-42; discussion S59-62.

9. Bhuta T, Ohlsson A. Systematic review and meta-analysis of early postnatal dexamethasone for prevention of chronic lung disease. *Arch Dis Child Fetal Neonatal Ed.* 1998;79(1):F26-33.

10. Halliday HL, Ehrenkranz RA, Doyle LW. Moderately early (7–14 days) postnatal corticosteroids for preventing chronic lung disease in preterm infants. *Cochrane Database Syst Rev.* 2003;(1):CD001144.

11. Yeh TF, et al. Early dexamethasone therapy in preterm infants: a follow-up study. *Pediatrics.* 1998;101(5):E7.

12. O'Shea TM, Washburn LK, Nixon PA, Goldstein DJ. Follow-up of a randomized, placebo-controlled trial of dexamethasone to decrease the duration of ventilator dependency in very low birth weight infants: neurodevelopmental outcomes at 4 to 11 years of age. *Pediatrics.* 2007;120(3):594-602.

13. Roberts R, Rodriguez W, Murphy D, Crescenzi T. Pediatric drug labeling: improving the safety and efficacy of pediatric therapies. *JAMA.* 2003;290(7): 905-911.

14. Giacoia GP, Birenbaum DL, Sachs HC, Mattison DR. The newborn drug development initiative. *Pediatrics.* 2006;117(3 Pt 2):S1-8.

15. Giacoia GP, Mattison DR. Selected proceedings of the NICHD/FDA newborn drug development initiative: Part II. *Clin Ther.* 2006;28(9):1337-1341.

16. Steinbrook R. Testing medications in children. *N Engl J Med.* 2002;347(18): 1462-1470.

17. Novak E, Allen PJ. Prescribing medications in pediatrics: concerns regarding FDA approval and pharmacokinetics. *Pediatr Nurs.* 2007;33(1):64-70.

18. Smith PB, et al. Pharmacokinetics of an elevated dosage of micafungin in premature neonates. *Pediatr Infect Dis J.* 2009;28(5):412-415.

19. Benjamin DK Jr, et al. Safety and pharmacokinetics of repeat-dose micafungin in young infants. *Clin Pharmacol Ther.* 2010;87(1):93-99.

20. Hope WW, et al. Population pharmacokinetics of micafungin in neonates and young infants. *Antimicrob Agents Chemother.* 2010;54(6):2633-2637.

21. Rodbro P, Krasilnikoff PA, Christiansen PM. Parietal cell secretory function in early childhood. *Scand J Gastroenterol.* 1967;2(3):209-213.

22. Agunod M, Yamaguchi N, Lopez R, Luhby AL, Glass GB. Correlative study of hydrochloric acid, pepsin, and intrinsic factor secretion in newborns and infants. *Am J Dig Dis.* 1969;14(6):400-414.

23. Kearns GL, et al. Developmental pharmacology–drug disposition, action, and therapy in infants and children. *N Engl J Med.* 2003;349(12):1157-1167.

24. Ittmann PI, Amarnath R, Berseth CL. Maturation of antroduodenal motor activity in preterm and term infants. *Dig Dis Sci.* 1992;37(1):14-19.

25. Heimann G. Enteral absorption and bioavailability in children in relation to age. *Eur J Clin Pharmacol.* 1980;18(1):43-50.

26. Giacoia GP, Mattison DR. Newborns and drug studies: the NICHD/FDA newborn drug development initiative. *Clin Ther.* 2005;27(6):796-813.

27. Yokoi T. Essentials for starting a pediatric clinical study (1): pharmacokinetics in children. *J Toxicol Sci.* 2009;34 (suppl) 2:SP307-312.

28. Ehrnebo M, Agurell S, Jalling B, Boréus LO. Age differences in drug binding by plasma proteins: studies on human foetuses, neonates and adults. *Eur J Clin Pharmacol.* 1971;3(4):189-193.

29. Shaddy RE, Denne SC. Clinical report–guidelines for the ethical conduct of studies to evaluate drugs in pediatric populations. *Pediatrics.* 2010;125(4): 850-860.

30. Koren G. Healthy children as subjects in pharmaceutical research. *Theor Med Bioeth.* 2003;24(2):149-159.

31. Department of Health and Human Services. 45 CFR Part 46 Protection of Human Subjects: Subpart D. Additional Protections for Children Involved as Subjects in Research. 2009. http://www.hhs.gov/ohrp/humansubjects/guidance/45cfr46.html#subpartd. Accessed April 24, 2012.

32. Rosenfield RL. Improving balance in regulatory oversight of research in children and adolescents: a clinical investigator's perspective. *Ann N Y Acad Sci.* 2008;1135:287-295.

33. Wade KC, et al. Population pharmacokinetics of fluconazole in young infants. *Antimicrob Agents Chemother.* 2008;52(11):4043-4049.

34. Aarons L. Population pharmacokinetics: theory and practice. *Br J Clin Pharmacol.* 1991;32(6):669-670.
35. Spooner N, Lad R, Barfield M. Dried blood spots as a sample collection technique for the determination of pharmacokinetics in clinical studies: considerations for the validation of a quantitative bioanalytical method. *Anal Chem.* 2009;81(4):1557-1563.
36. Anon. Informed consent elements. Final rule. *Fed Regist.* 2011;76(2): 256-270.
37. Li JS, et al. Economic return of clinical trials performed under the pediatric exclusivity program. *JAMA.* 2007;297(5):480-488.
38. US Food and Drug Administration. New Pediatric Labeling Information Database. http://www.accessdata.fda.gov/scripts/sda/sdNavigation.cfm?sd= labelingdatabase. Accessed April 4, 2012.
39. Salazar JC. Pediatric clinical trial experience: government, child, parent and physician's perspective. *Pediatr Infect Dis J.* 2003;22(12):1124-1127.
40. Simone JV, Lyons J. Superior cancer survival in children compared to adults: a superior system of cancer care? Background paper for National Cancer Policy Board, Institute of Medicine. *Docstoc.com.* 1998. http://www.docstoc.com/docs/69303193/Superior-Cancer-Survival-in-Children-Compared-to-Adults–A. Accessed April 24, 2012.
41. American Cancer Society. Cancer Facts & Figures—2012. 2012. http://www.cancer.org/Research/CancerFactsFigures/ACSPC-031941. Accessed April 24, 2012.

Observational Research

CHAPTER TEN

Observational Research

Michaela A. Dinan

Clinical research can be broadly divided into two subsets: experimental research and observational research. The vast majority of new medical treatments and technologies are tested through experimental or interventional research, often in the form of randomized trials, before they are adopted into clinical use. In contrast, observational studies are primarily conducted on technologies after they have already been adopted and are being implemented in some sector of the healthcare community. Observational research occupies a critical niche within healthcare research that is complementary to experimental studies. Understanding the relative strengths, weaknesses, similarities, and differences between observational and experimental research is critical to accurately interpreting clinical research.

A WORKING DEFINITION OF OBSERVATIONAL RESEARCH

Observational research is a research in which the investigator cannot control the assignment of treatment to subjects because the participants or conditions are not being directly assigned by the researcher. Observational research examines predetermined treatments, interventions, and policies and their effects. In practical terms, observational comparative effectiveness research (CER) is typically conducted within one of two settings, either within registries or as subgroup analyses within randomized clinical trials. Registries are generally created with a specific disease, treatment, or population of interest, and can occur within a specific institution, network of institutions, or geographic region within which clinically relevant outcomes are recorded. Subgroup analyses within clinical trials include any subset for which patients are not randomly assigned.

Because subgroups are not randomly assigned, subgroup analyses share all the strengths and weaknesses of conventional observational studies, such as confounding and multiple hypotheses testing, and provide a similar level of evidence.

In contrast to observational research, researchers in experimental studies directly manipulate or assign participants to different interventions or environments. A third type of research involves descriptive studies, which are conducted without a treatment and are neither experimental nor observational (1). This type of research is used in the initial exploration and characterization of a healthcare issue. Descriptive studies play no direct role in CER, whereas experimental and observational studies are important in both developmental and CER.

STRENGTHS AND WEAKNESSES OF OBSERVATIONAL RESEARCH WITHIN COMPARATIVE EFFECTIVENESS RESEARCH

Recent focus on the importance of CER was reinvigorated with passage of the Patient Protection and Affordable Care Act (PPACA) in 2010 (2). From a practical research standpoint, this emphasis on CER makes it important to define and understand observational research within the context of CER.

The Agency for Healthcare Research and Quality (AHRQ), the lead federal agency responsible for improving healthcare quality in the United States, defines CER as research that provides "evidence on the effectiveness, benefits, and harms of different treatment options" (3). This evidence is generated via comparative studies of drugs, medical devices, tests, surgeries, or ways to deliver health care. We find such evidence in one of two ways: through experimental studies or through observational studies. Each of these approaches has different strengths and weaknesses, and each uses both overlapping and distinct methods.

In a CER context, the strength of experimental studies is that they provide the strongest evaluation or validation of a specific, well-defined intervention or treatment. In particular, experimental studies provide the highest level of evidence for evaluating new therapies, which includes the current "gold standard" in CER—the randomized controlled trial (RCT). In recent years, several examples have arisen in which observational studies have been confounded by selection bias, which have later been contradicted by RCTs (Table 10–1).

TABLE 10–1

Examples of randomized controlled trials contradicting observational data

Clinical question	Observational studies	Randomized controlled trial	Insight from RCTs
Does hormone replacement therapy provide cardiovascular protection for women?	>30 studies recommending cardioprotective benefit	HERS (4): • No difference in cardiovascular events • Significant increase in venous thromboembolic events • Significant decrease in fractures	• Prevalent user bias • Women who elected to use hormone therapy were healthier overall
Does vitamin B12 and folate supplementation reduce cardiovascular risk?	>100 observational studies finding improved outcomes and homocysteine reduction	SEARCH (5): • 12,064 survivors of MI randomized to receive folate and vitamin B12 and followed for 6.7 years • Vascular event rates of 25.5% in treatment arm versus 24.8% in placebo arm ($P = 0.28$)	• Prevalent user bias • People who elected to use supplementation were more likely healthier overall

HERS, Heart Estrogen–Progestin Study; MI, myocardial infarction; SEARCH, Study of the Effectiveness of Additional Reductions in Cholesterol and Homocysteine.

One of the best-known examples of this is the effect of hormone replacement therapy on women's health. Numerous observational studies had shown a cardioprotective benefit of this therapy against heart attack and stroke in women. However, a large randomized clinical trial later showed that women randomized to receive hormone therapy showed no difference in cardiovascular events, a reduced fracture risk, and significant increases in venous clot formation and embolic events (4). Another example is the concept that vitamin B12 and folate supplementation could reduce the risk of major coronary events. This hypothesis was initially supported by numerous observational data but was later refuted by the randomized Study of the Effectiveness of Additional Reductions in Cholesterol and Homocysteine (SEARCH) (5).

In both cases, the conclusion was that selection bias was likely confounding the results of observational studies. Women receiving hormone therapy appeared to differ systematically from women who were not receiving hormone therapy (prevalent user bias), and the previously observed association between hormone therapy and cardioprotection likely resulted from confounding by overall improved access to health care, patient demographics, and other unobserved phenomena associated with therapy and improved cardiovascular health. The use of hormone therapy in women and its effects on cardioprotection remain actively debated topics; nonetheless, they serve as important examples of discrepancies between observational studies and RCTs.

The strength of the experimental study—evaluation of a specific, controllable treatment, or exposure—is also responsible for its key weakness: being difficult, impractical, or even impossible to conduct in complex, poorly defined, or poorly controlled situations. This limitation becomes particularly apparent in complex or organization-level studies of health-care systems, in unpredictable or emergency settings, and when examining factors that cannot be assigned for either ethical or practical reasons, such as patient demographics, genotypes, social factors, or disease status. A further area for caution with regard to experimental studies stems from the fact that they take place in tightly controlled clinical settings. An intervention tested by experts in tertiary-care academic medical centers might lack generalizability (i.e., not be applicable to general clinical practice or the general patient population), if the trial setting differs significantly from conditions in actual practice (Table 10–2).

For example, the Can Rapid risk stratification of Unstable angina patients Suppress ADverse outcomes with Early implementation of the ACC/AHA guidelines? (CRUSADE) registry of more 400 emergency departments and medical centers was designed to examine actual practices regarding management of patients with non-ST-segment elevation myocardial infarction (NSTEMI). The investigators observed an inpatient mortality rate of ~5% (6), roughly two to three times greater than the rates observed in three randomized clinical trials of NSTEMI treatments (7–9). This same analysis showed that in clinical practice, guideline adherence was not uniform and substantially affected patient outcomes; a 10% increase in guideline adherence was associated with a 10% relative decrease in mortality (6). In another example, implantation of cardiac defibrillators occurs more often

TABLE 10–2

Examples of observational studies providing insight unavailable through randomized trials

Clinical question	Observational studies	Randomized controlled trial(s)	Insight from observational studies
ACS mortality risk	CRUSADE registry of ~180,000 patients (6) • 5% mortality after ACS	PURSUIT (7), CURE (8), SYNERGY (9) • Lower rates of comorbidities (age, diabetes, kidney disease) and prior heart disease (heart failure, previous MI): • 1–2% mortality after ACS	Clinical trial populations are often healthier than patients in general clinical practice
Receipt of cardiac defibrillators	Odds ratio versus white men (10): • Black men: 0.73 • White women: 0.62 • Black women: 0.54	• Inequitable care not captured • Would be unethical within an RCT to mirror unequal treatment observed in actual practice	In general clinical practice, patient sex and race affect treatment
Early cardiac catheterization	• Patients with highest risk of disease least likely to be catheterized (11)	• Actual clinical practice not captured • Would be unethical within an RCT to deny treatment to highest-risk patients	In general clinical practice, high-risk patients are least likely to receive care
Guideline adherence after ACS	10% increase in guideline adherence associated with 10% reduced mortality (6)	• Variation in guideline adherence not captured • Would be unethical within an RCT to not follow guidelines	In general clinical practice, compliance with guidelines is not uniform or 100%
Medication adherence after hospital discharge	Decreased treatment adherence within 6 months after discharge (12)	• Clinical trials stop at discharge • Unable to follow-up patients indefinitely within RCTs due to feasibility and costs	Patient outcomes are often affected by phenomena outside trial observation windows

ACS, acute coronary syndrome; MI, myocardial infarction; RCT, randomized clinical trial.

in white men than in other demographics, with black women being about half as likely as to receive the same care (10). Finally, patients who are at highest risk of having an acute coronary event appear to be least likely in practice to undergo cardiac catheterization (11). The general conclusion to keep in mind when interpreting randomized trials, then, is that such trials often do not reflect general practice; patients seen in actual practice can be older, have more comorbid conditions, and not receive the standard of care that would be expected from academic medical centers. This is especially true for long-term therapies after discharge. Clinical trials in acute coronary syndromes typically stop at hospital discharge, even though observational studies of patient outcomes after hospitalization show that patients often stop taking their medications within 6 months after discharge (12).

Finally, experimental studies are costly in terms of both time and resources—a single trial can easily cost millions of dollars, take years to complete, and involve large numbers of clinical, administrative, and research personnel.

The observational approach to CER provides a complementary approach to randomized trials, with a different set of strengths and weaknesses. The strengths of observational research lie in the fact that it can be conveniently applied to actual practice patterns and any naturally (or unnaturally) occurring phenomenon. It is not limited to artificial, relatively limited, controlled research settings that may have questionable generalizability. Observational studies can reflect how an intervention is truly being used in general medical practice. In addition to the theoretical advantage of more generalized inferences, observational studies offer several practical advantages. They are typically much less expensive and easier to conduct with regard to practical, clinical, and ethical issues. As a result, they typically involve much larger sample sizes, which allow for increased statistical power. With the appropriate dataset, entire populations can be directly studied, such as through the use of registries or census data.

The key weakness of observational studies is that, by definition, they cannot randomly (or otherwise) assign an intervention to study participants. Because assignment of treatment is not under the control of the investigator, any observational study will always have the potential for confounding and thus drawing incorrect inferences from a study. Patients or study participants who receive an intervention can be and most often are systematically different from patients who do not receive the intervention. New investigational interventions are typically applied to patients for whom standard care has failed, often selecting for sick patients. On the other hand, new investigational tools are often applied only to patients who are healthier and believed to stand a chance of tolerating a new therapy. Unfortunately, there is always a potential for confounding in any observational study, making correct study design and accurate interpretation of paramount importance.

OBSERVATIONAL RESEARCH IN THE HIERARCHY OF EVIDENCE

The two main benefits of observational studies over experimental studies, feasibility and generalizability, are balanced by their critical weakness, the potential for confounding. As a result, observational studies are generally considered a lower standard of evidence with regard to CER.

In general, CER is used to determine the relative effectiveness of one intervention versus another. When evaluating the efficacy of potential treatments, the randomized, double-blind, placebo-controlled trial is considered the strongest or highest level of evidence that an intervention is better than either a placebo or an alternative therapy (Figure 10–1) (13).

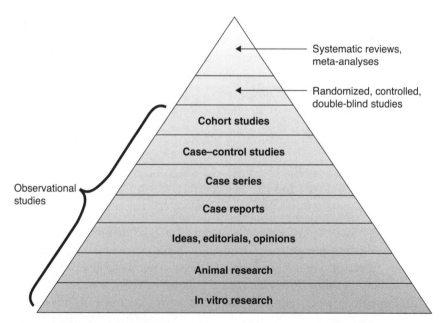

FIGURE 10–1. Hierarchy of clinical evidence. Adapted, with permission, from SUNY Downstate Medical Center, Medical Library of Brooklyn. Evidence Based Medicine Course. A Guide to Research Methods: The Evidence Pyramid. 2004. http://library.downstate.edu/EBM2/2100.htm. Accessed May 4, 2012.

There are several reasons for this, the most important of which is the fact that randomization removes the potential for confounding of the perceived effects of the intervention. Other benefits of the randomized, controlled, double-blind trial come from blinding of the study personnel to avoid evaluator bias and using a placebo to provide an accurate and fair control reference. Sometimes blinding is not used because it is inconvenient or impossible to blind either subjects or investigators—for example, when one treatment group is easily identified because its patients receive surgery or drugs that carry significant side effects. Blinding is important when outcomes are subjective, but it is less of an issue when "hard" end points are being studied (death, organ failure, etc.). Such outcomes are unlikely to be affected by the investigator's opinion or mindset.

Evidence hierarchies such as the one depicted in Figure 10–1 often refer to the evaluation of well-defined interventions in which the goal is to evaluate whether an intervention improves a specific outcome. Some researchers have suggested that different hierarchies should be used depending on the research goal; for example, when exploring complex, new, or relatively unknown phenomena, observational or even anecdotal studies can serve as initial steps in gaining knowledge and directing future study. Some investigators and researchers are split between the experimental and observational mindsets, but regardless of one's background, it is important to appreciate the strengths and weaknesses of each. In the end, it may be best to consider all available evidence from different approaches. In CER, both experimental and observational studies are trying to assess the same thing—causality of an intervention (14).

SUBSETS OF OBSERVATIONAL RESEARCH WITHIN HEALTH CARE

In practice, observational studies of health often fall into one of three areas within healthcare research: epidemiology, health economics, and health services research. Distinctions among these areas have developed over time, largely because different research questions require different types of data, methods, and background knowledge to be successfully answered. Epidemiology has evolved around naturally occurring exposures, interventions, or differences that are distributed by forces outside the healthcare system, whereas health services research tends to focus on those directly or indirectly caused by a healthcare system. Health services researchers often further define their interests in quality, access, or costs. Health economics focuses on this last topic, examining the economics of healthcare costs, resource allocation, and business models of health care. Although each of these areas has developed a subject-specific set of knowledge, methods, data, and perspectives, these types of studies can overlap substantially. As with all observational research, they are interested in inferring causality so that we can learn something about health.

Epidemiology

Several formal definitions are used to describe epidemiology. One of the most useful ways to define epidemiology functionally is by examining its word origin. "Epi" and "dem" come from the Greek for "upon" and "people," respectively, to yield the definition "upon the people." This probably best describes what makes epidemiology unique as a field within health research: epidemiology is the study of exposures or traits placed "upon the people" by nature or outside forces, usually in contrast to exposures chosen by or given to the people via policy, healthcare providers, or other direct intention.

Epidemiological work in health services research tends to focus on exposures or other interventions that cannot be controlled or for which there is not sufficient money, interest, time, or effort to control in a formal trial. No randomized trial has been conducted to show that smoking causes heart or lung disease, yet the association of smoking with these diseases, particularly lung cancer, makes smoking the most potent modifiable risk factor in health care to date. Effects of lead poisoning on child development, identification of carcinogens, the interplay between the environment and asthma, and the association of diet and lifestyle choices with health are all important areas of health knowledge that have been advanced through epidemiological studies.

Health Services Research

Health services research as defined by Rosenbaum (1) is an "applied multidisciplinary field that uses scientific inquiry to produce knowledge about the resources, provisions, organizing, financing, and policies of health services at the population level." Within the "iron triangle of health care"—quality, access, and costs—health services research tends to focus more on quality and access than on economics, but this is largely an artificial distinction caused by differences in methods. Health services research finds its use in areas of health care where the intervention of interest cannot feasibly be manipulated, such as demographics or distance to care, and it is critical for examining and guiding healthcare policy.

Examples of health services research include analyses of large healthcare systems' practices or health policy changes. Health services research can be used to analyze the effects of national, state, or local government policies, differences between health systems, and effects of sociodemographics on care, health disparities, or practice patterns. These types of studies are numerous; they have been used to investigate how Medicare changes in reimbursement affect quality of care, to assess the adoption of new medical technology in general use, and to identify consistent associations between race and disparate health outcomes.

Health Economics

The economics of healthcare focus on costs, where costs can be measured in terms of money, time, resource use, quality of life, or some combination of these. Health economics research can be conducted on a global, national, regional, or institutional scale, depending on the stakeholders involved and the question being investigated. These studies are often observational; for example, they can be conducted after implementing a change in medical practice to evaluate its financial implications and long-term sustainability.

The most readily available examples of health economics research are typically those that examine the costs of health care and related expenses. Such research can focus within a healthcare entity to examine work-time-flow efficiency, billing practices, revenue generation, and effects of intramural policies. More societally focused examples of health economics research include population-level budgeting and cost-effectiveness analyses. For example, in April 2012, Medicare released its annual Trustees Report, which uses actuarial spending trends to calculate when Medicare will no longer be solvent under current practices (15). Cost-effectiveness analyses serve to assess and provide a common denominator regarding how much a group is willing to pay for a certain amount of benefit. For example, in the United States, treatments are generally considered to be reasonably cost-effective at a cost of $50,000 per quality-adjusted year of life (QALY) (16). Treatments or interventions that are the most cost-effective will, in theory, be adopted most readily and widely.

Commonalities Among Epidemiology, Health Services Research, and Health Economics

Although the focuses of specific fields differ within observational studies of health, these disciplines also have many similarities and overlapping features (17,18). All observational research seeks to establish causality (14) and inform practice. The same basic conceptual approach is used—a treatment, intervention, or exposure of interest is selected; the relevant outcome is identified; the outcome of the study is assessed by statistical analysis; and the magnitude of effect is used to assess implications. Similar challenges are faced in all observational research, including a potential for misinterpretation and poor study design. Again, most studies use the same basic concepts, even if they use different language (19). For example, the primary outcome of a study might be referred to as the *dependent variable* in some studies versus the *primary end point* in others. Observational research, regardless of the field, still generally uses the same statistical methods, with the only real difference being a focused appreciation for practical concerns (20).

CONCLUSION

Observational research is research in which the assignment of treatment to subjects is not directly assigned. This typically occurs within the context of disease or treatment registries or in nonrandomized subgroup analyses within randomized clinical trials. The key strength of observational studies is that they can assess care as it is delivered in clinical practice, not in the carefully controlled settings of randomized controlled trials. The caution in using observational studies comes from their inability to remove treatment bias and confounders, which can lead to spurious results. In the end, observational research forms a key component of health outcomes research that must be incorporated into CER, to fully understand how treatments studied under ideal circumstances will translate when applied to general practice.

REFERENCES

1. Rosenbaum PR. *Observational Studies*. 2nd ed. New York, NY: Springer-Verlag; 2010.
2. U.S. Congress. *Patient Protection and Affordable Care Act*. 2010. http://www.gpo.gov/fdsys/pkg/PLAW-111publ148/content-detail.html. Accessed May 4, 2012.

3. Agency for Healthcare Research and Quality. What Is Comparative Effectiveness Research. http://effectivehealthcare.ahrq.gov/index.cfm/what-is-comparative-effectiveness-research1/. Accessed May 4, 2012.

4. Hulley S, et al. Randomized trial of estrogen plus progestin for secondary prevention of coronary heart disease in postmenopausal women. Heart and Estrogen/progestin Replacement Study (HERS) Research Group. *JAMA*. 1998;280(7):605-613.

5. Armitage JM, et al. Effects of homocysteine-lowering with folic acid plus vitamin B12 vs placebo on mortality and major morbidity in myocardial infarction survivors: a randomized trial. *JAMA*. 2010;303(24):2486-2494.

6. Peterson ED, et al. Association between hospital process performance and outcomes among patients with acute coronary syndromes. *JAMA*. 2006;295 (16):1912-1920.

7. The PURSUIT Trial Investigators. Inhibition of platelet glycoprotein IIb/IIIa with eptifibatide in patients with acute coronary syndromes. *N Engl J Med*. 1998;339(7):436-443.

8. Yusuf S, et al. Effects of clopidogrel in addition to aspirin in patients with acute coronary syndromes without ST-segment elevation. *N Engl J Med*. 2001;345(7):494-502.

9. Ferguson JJ, et al. Enoxaparin vs unfractionated heparin in high-risk patients with non-ST-segment elevation acute coronary syndromes managed with an intended early invasive strategy: primary results of the SYNERGY randomized trial. *JAMA*. 2004;292(1):45-54.

10. Hernandez AF, et al. Sex and racial differences in the use of implantable cardioverter-defibrillators among patients hospitalized with heart failure. *JAMA*. 2007;298(13):1525-1532.

11. Tricoci P, et al. Temporal trends in the use of early cardiac catheterization in patients with non-ST-segment elevation acute coronary syndromes (results from CRUSADE). *Am J Cardiol*. 2006;98(9):1172-1176.

12. Eagle KA, et al. Adherence to evidence-based therapies after discharge for acute coronary syndromes: an ongoing prospective, observational study. *Am J Med*. 2004;117(2):73-81.

13. SUNY Downstate Medical Center, Medical Library of Brooklyn. Evidence Based Medicine Course. A Guide to Research Methods: The Evidence Pyramid. 2004. http://library.downstate.edu/EBM2/2100.htm. Accessed May 4, 2012.

14. Dowd BE. Separated at birth: statisticians, social scientists, and causality in health services research. *Health Serv Res*. 2011;46(2):397-420.

15. Boards of Trustees, Federal Hospital Insurance and Federal Supplementary Medical Insurance Trust Funds. 2012 Annual report of the Boards of Trustees of the Federal Hospital Insurance and Federal Supplementary Medical Insurance Trust Funds. 2012. https://www.cms.gov/Research-Statistics-Data-and-Systems/Statistics-Trends-and-Reports/ReportsTrustFunds/Downloads/TR2012.pdf. Accessed May 4, 2012.

16. Ubel PA, Hirth RA, Chernew ME, Fendrick AM. What is the price of life and why doesn't it increase at the rate of inflation? *Arch Intern Med.* 2003; 163(14):1637-1641.

17. Vandenbroucke JP. Observational research, randomised trials, and two views of medical science. *PLoS Med.* 2008;5(3):e67.

18. Berwick DM. The science of improvement. *JAMA.* 2008;299(10):1182-1184.

19. Maciejewski ML, Weaver EM, Hebert PL. Synonyms in health services research methodology. *Med Care Res Rev.* 2011;68(2):156-176.

20. Kennedy PE. *A Guide to Econometrics.* 5th ed. Cambridge, MA: MIT Press; 2003.

CHAPTER ELEVEN

Data Resources

Ying Xian

This chapter reviews various data sources available for observational research, examines their strengths and limitations, and identifies opportunities for further improving observational databases by integrating data collected from different sources. The focus is on observational research using existing databases.

CLINICAL REGISTRIES

Clinical registries have an important role in observational research. In this section, we first review an array of the available clinical registries that are closely or broadly relevant to cardiovascular disease (Table 11–1). We then summarize the strengths and limitations of clinical registries for observational study.

American Heart Association— Get With The Guidelines

Get With The Guidelines® (GWTG) is a national cardiovascular disease registry and quality improvement program developed by the American Heart Association (AHA) and American Stroke Association. The GWTG registry includes three modules—one each for coronary artery disease, heart failure, and stroke (1)—and one outpatient program (2). GWTG uses a Web-based patient management tool (Outcomes, Cambridge, MA) to abstract detailed clinical data, including patient demographics, medical history, symptoms on arrival, in-hospital treatment and events, contraindications to medications, laboratory findings, discharge treatment and counseling, and patient disposition from more than 381,000 patients in the heart failure module and more than 1,000,000 patients in the stroke module. In 2008, the coronary disease module was merged with the

TABLE 11–1
Evolution of cardiovascular clinical registries

Database	Size	Examples
Clinicians' own experiences	10–100s	Osler, Harvey
Single center databases	1000–10,000s	Duke Databank for Cardiovascular Diseases Emory Cardiac Database
Epidemiological cohorts	10,000s	National Heart, Lung, and Blood Institute Dynamic Registry
National registries	Millions	American Heart Association Get With The Guidelines American College of Cardiology National Cardiovascular Data Registry Society of Thoracic Surgeons National Database
Global registries	Potentially billions	Global Registry of Acute Coronary Events (GRACE) ProspeCtive observational LongitudinAl RegIstry oF patients with stable coronary arterY disease (CLARIFY)

American College of Cardiology (ACC) Acute Coronary Treatment and Intervention Outcomes Network (ACTION®) registry to form the National Cardiovascular Data Registry (NCDR) ACTION Registry–GWTG, which has become the most comprehensive data source for acute coronary syndromes in the United States (3). In 2011, the GWTG outpatient program was expanded to become The Guideline Advantage™, in collaboration with the American Cancer Society and American Diabetes Association (2).

American College of Cardiology— National Cardiovascular Data Registry

This is a comprehensive outcomes-based quality improvement program operated by the ACC since 1997 (4). More than 2,200 hospitals participate in the NCDR across the United States. The NCDR includes the outpatient Practice INNovation And CLinical Excellence (PINNACLE) registry, with more than 1.5 million records, and various hospital-based registries, including ACTION Registry–GWTG, for patients with high-risk myocardial infarction; CathPCI, for cardiac catheterizations and percutaneous coronary intervention procedures; the ICD Registry, for tracking implantable cardioverter defibrillator procedures; the CARE Registry, for carotid artery stenting and endarterectomy; and the IMPACT registry, for pediatric and adult patients with congenital heart disease who are undergoing diagnostic catheterization and interventions.

CRUSADE

Can Rapid risk stratification of Unstable patients with angina Suppress ADverse outcomes with Early implementation of the ACC/AHA guidelines? (CRUSADE) is a clinical registry of more than 200,000 patients with acute coronary syndromes at 600 hospitals in the United States (5). Data collected include patient risk factors, presenting symptoms, use of medications/invasive procedures, and in-hospital clinical outcomes focused on the ACC/AHA guidelines.

Society of Thoracic Surgeons— Adult Cardiac Surgery Database

This is the largest cardiothoracic surgery quality improvement and outcomes database in the world (6). The society provides clinical details and outcomes for more than 4.3 million coronary artery bypass graft surgeries and valvular and other cardiac procedures from 1,014 participating sites in the United States.

ADHERE

The Acute Decompensated Heart failurE national REgistry (ADHERE) is an industry-sponsored, multicenter, national registry evaluating the characteristics, management, and clinical outcomes of patients hospitalized with acute decompensated heart failure (7). More than 150,000 patients from 300 community and academic centers in the United States were enrolled between 2001 and 2006.

OPTIMIZE-HF

The Organized Program To Initiate life-saving treatMent In hospitaliZEd patients with Heart Failure (OPTIMIZE- HF) is a national registry designed to evaluate and improve guideline adherence among hospitalized patients with heart failure (8). Unlike ADHERE and many other clinical registries reporting only in-hospital events, OPTIMIZE-HF captures outcomes data at 60 and 90 days after discharge for selected patients (10%). The OPTI-MIZE-HF project transitioned to GWTG-HF in 2005.

PREMIER, TRIUMPH

The Prospective Registry Evaluating Myocardial Infarction: Event and Recovery (PREMIER) (9) and Translational Research Investigating Underlying disparities in acute Myocardial infarction Patients' Health status (TRIUMPH) (10) are prospective multicenter registries of 7000 patients with acute myocardial infarction (2,500 in PREMIER and 4,500 in TRIUMPH). A distinct feature of PREMIER and TRIUMPH is that patient-centered outcome measures, including symptoms, functional status, and quality of life, are collected at 1, 6, and 12 months after the index hospitalization.

Strengths and Limitations of Clinical Registries

Among the most important strengths of clinical registries are broader population coverage, solid exposure and outcomes measures, and rich clinical data available to adjust for confounding variables. Clinical registries tend to include a large number of patients; registry-based findings therefore can be more generalizable to a wide range of patients than can those from randomized controlled trials (RCTs), which contain more homogenous populations in ideal situations. Exposure/treatment and outcomes/effectiveness are better defined in a registry than in administrative data. Additionally, rich clinical information, such as risk factors and comorbid conditions, can be used to build precise risk-adjustment models. Finally, clinical registries provide an opportunity to evaluate the effectiveness of interventions in cases in which randomization is unethical or impractical (e.g., studies of surgical procedures).

Despite the clear strengths of clinical registries, several limitations should be noted. Unlike in clinical trials, in which patients are randomized to either a treatment or a control arm, outcomes assessment using registry data can be subject to selection bias. In addition, registries are often limited in terms of their targeted population. Unlike hospital administrative data, a clinical registry often focuses on certain diseases and conditions. For instance, it is unrealistic to use a stroke registry for cancer research. Another drawback of many clinical registries has been the lack of follow-up data beyond hospital discharge or the acute episode of care. Knowledge obtained in hospital may not be applicable to intermediate or long-term outcomes. Methods have been developed to address this limitation by linking clinical registry data with external data sources. These strategies are discussed later in this chapter.

ADMINISTRATIVE DATA

Administrative data are typically generated and gathered for some administrative purpose such as billing upon hospital discharge or provision of other health services. These data often include patient demographics, disease diagnoses, and medications or procedures received, allowing their use for clinical research as well. There is an increasing popularity in using large administrative datasets for observational study and comparative effectiveness research (CER). Among all data sources, administrative data have perhaps the broadest population coverage, an attribute especially appealing to CER. For example, Medicare (Parts A and B) alone was providing health care to more than 43 million people as of July 2010, including more than 36 million aged 65 or older (11).

Medicare Datasets

Medicare datasets contain data for institutional claims (inpatient, outpatient, skilled nursing facility, hospice, or home health agency) and noninstitutional claims (physician and durable medical equipment providers) (12). The 5% sample is created from the 100% Denominator file based on the beneficiary's Health Insurance Claim (HIC) number. Medicare claims data do not contain laboratory results or medication information.

The Medicare Denominator File contains demographics that include beneficiary unique identifier, state, county, ZIP code, date of birth, sex, race, date of death, program eligibility, and enrollment information (13).

The Medicare Part D File contains information about prescriptions that beneficiaries had filled under Medicare Part D. As of 2008, nearly 25 million Medicare beneficiaries were enrolled in Medicare Part D plans.

These data can be linked with Medicare physician and hospital claims under Parts A and B of the program and can serve as a rich data source to describe medication use patterns, health outcomes, and adverse events among aged and disabled Medicare beneficiaries (9).

The Medicare Provider Analysis and Review File (MedPAR) contains the accumulated claims for services provided to a beneficiary from the time of inpatient hospital admission to discharge home or to a skilled nursing facility. It allows tracking of inpatient hospitalizations and patterns of care over time (14).

The Medicare Current Beneficiary Survey (MCBS) is a nationally representative survey of the Medicare population regarding their health status and functioning, healthcare use and expenditures, health insurance coverage, and sociodemographic characteristics. It includes oversampled aged, disabled, and institutionalized beneficiaries (15).

The Medicaid Analytic eXtract (MAX), formerly known as the State Medicaid Research Files (SMRFs), is a set of person-level data files containing information on Medicaid eligibility, enrollment status, demographic data, utilization summary, inpatient care, long-term care, medication claims, and claims for all noninstitutional Medicaid services (16).

US Department of Veterans Affairs (VA)
Administrative Datasets

The VA Patient Treatment File contains records for all inpatient care received by all covered persons at VA care facilities. Information collected includes demographics, diagnoses, procedures, and summary information for each episode of care (17).

The VA Outpatient Clinic File contains records for all outpatient care received by all covered persons from 1980 to the present (17).

The VA Pharmacy Benefits Management Services Database contains all prescriptions dispensed within the VA health system from 1999 to the present (18).

VA Decision Support System (DSS) Data Extracts contain cost and use information on inpatient and outpatient laboratory testing, prescription medications, radiological procedures, and demographics for all VA patients (19). Unlike other administrative data, results for a specific list of laboratory tests are included in the DSS.

The VA Vital Status File (VSF) contains the date of death information for all veterans who received VA care after 1992, who were enrolled in the VA, or who received compensation or pension benefits from the VA after 2002 (20).

Agency for Healthcare Research and Quality

The Health Care Cost and Utilization Project (HCUP) includes the largest collection of hospital care data in the United States (21). It includes the Nationwide Inpatient Sample (NIS) and State Inpatient Databases (SID). The NIS includes more than 100 clinical and nonclinical data elements for each inpatient stay from a stratified sample of about 20% of community hospitals across the country. Information includes patient demographics, admission and discharge status, principal and up to 30 secondary diagnosis codes, principal and secondary procedure codes, length of stay, and total charges. The SID contains similar data elements but includes 100% inpatient discharge records from participating states. Both the NIS and SID contain hospital identifiers that permit linkage with the American Hospital Association Annual Survey data and county identifiers for linkage to the Area Resource File.

The Medical Expenditure Panel Survey (MEPS) is a set of nationally representative surveys of healthcare use, expenditures, sources of payment, health insurance coverage, and health status for noninstitutionalized Americans (22). A unique feature of MEPS is that it includes data on traditionally underrepresented populations such as poor, older, minority, and uninsured citizens.

Commercial Insurance Claims

The MarketScan Commercial Claims and Encounters database from Thomson Reuters (Healthcare) Inc. contains fully integrated, de-identified, person-specific data on enrollment, clinical use, and expenditures across inpatient, outpatient laboratory, and outpatient prescriptions from about 100 commercial, Medicare supplemental, and Medicaid payers (23). MarketScan can be linked to track-detailed patient information across sites and types of providers and over time.

Kaiser Permanente is a large, integrated healthcare delivery system. Its electronic medical records, laboratory, and pharmacy databases include claims data for both inpatient and outpatient services (24).

Strengths and Limitations of Administrative Data

The main strength of administrative data is the broad coverage of populations. Findings from administrative databases can be easily implemented in real-world settings. Because most administrative datasets are relatively large, it is possible to focus on groups traditionally underrepresented in other data sources, such as racial/ethnic minority, female, and older patients. Moreover, administrative data are relatively more efficient to obtain because no additional primary data collection is needed. Importantly, many administrative data have common identifiers that make long-term follow-up possible.

Despite these strengths, administrative data can have major limitations. First and foremost, the data can be "dirty." Administrative data in general are gathered for the purpose of medical billing. Some data elements are likely to be more accurate than others. For instance, providers are not penalized for providing inaccurate information unless it is associated with medical payments. Second, compared with clinical trial and registry databases, important clinical details such as secondary diagnoses and procedures are often undercoded, making risk-adjustment difficult (25). Third, except for a few sources, many administrative databases do not contain laboratory and pharmacy data. Consequently, secondary data analyses using administrative data can seldom give a complete clinical picture.

TRIAL DATABASES

When talking about data sources for observational studies, people often think of clinical registries and hospital administrative data. However, observational studies also can be done with secondary use of existing data from clinical trials databases. For instance, researchers can transfer information from either the treatment or the control arm and evaluate it for purposes other than that specified in the original RCT design.

Because RCTs are generally accepted as the gold standard for clinical evidence, many attributes of a reliable and robust database for clinical research have been built into such study designs. For example, RCT databases contain well-delineated exposure measures, objective outcome assessments, rich clinical information, and few confounding variables. Despite these advantages, however, secondary analyses of trial data have the same limitations as do primary analyses of RCT data. For instance, RCTs are designed to evaluate the efficacy and safety of a treatment or intervention under ideal circumstances. Thus, the population included in an RCT is often narrowly selected, making the results not necessarily generalizable to patients who will eventually use the medication or treatment in real-world settings.

LINKING DATASETS—
OPPORTUNITIES AND CHALLENGES

Given the pros and cons of RCTs and registries, investigators have considered merging them, to create registry–trial hybrids for clinical research. The National Cardiovascular Research Infrastructure (NCRI) is a partnership between the American College of Cardiology Foundation (ACCF) and the Duke Clinical Research Institute (DCRI) to develop a multicenter translational research model based on the data-collection activities of the NCDR. The NCRI recruits registry sites as clinical trial participants, uses a standard registry data-collection system already in use by the hospitals, and adds additional data elements for the specific trials to the NCDR backbone. This creates an efficient clinical research platform for randomized clinical trials based on the existing registry.

The Study of Access site For Enhancement of Percutaneous Coronary Intervention (SAFE-PCI) for Women is a multicenter, randomized, open-label, active-control study comparing the efficacy and feasibility of the transradial approach versus the transfemoral approach to PCI in women (NCT01406236). It is one of the first proof-of-concept trials to use the NCRI. The study identifies sites within the NCDR system, and patients enrolled at participating sites are randomized to undergo either transfemoral or transradial PCI before diagnostic angiography. Data-collection efforts are further reduced by using the existing NCDR data-collection system. All these efforts improve operational efficiency in clinical trials.

Besides the integration of trials into ongoing registries, there is increasing interest in creating a linked claims–registry database, with rich clinical information as well as longitudinal outcome assessments, that takes advantage of the strengths of both databases and overcomes their limitations. The major challenge in linking different data sources is the availability of the identifying information in each dataset. Some databases contain standard personal identifiers such as patient name and Social Security number, making it possible to link a clinical registry directly with administrative data sources. However, many clinical registries do not collect or distribute unencrypted patient identifiers. Nevertheless, high-quality linkages can be made using various combinations of nonunique fields. Hammill et al. described a method of linking inpatient clinical registry data to Medicare claims data using indirect identifiers (26). They showed that by using a combination of indirect identifiers available in both datasets, such as admission date, discharge date, patient age or date of birth, and patient sex, a high-quality linked database can be created without requiring direct identifiers.

Linking clinical registries and administrative data overcomes the lack of clinical details in administrative databases and the absence of long-term assessments in registry data. Importantly, a linked dataset extends the applications of both data sources, provides a full picture of the care delivered, and approaches the ideal for assessing CER in real-world clinical practice. Linking clinical registry and administrative data also has limitations. Using indirect identifiers can cause inaccurate links between databases; thus, external validation is recommended if the data are available (27). In addition, linkage almost always limits the analysis population, which, in turn, raises concerns about the generalizability of the study findings.

In summary, various data sources, including clinical registries, hospital administrative data, and trial databases, are available for observational study. Researchers must evaluate the strengths versus limitations of each type to determine the most appropriate data source to answer their research questions.

REFERENCES

1. Hong Y, LaBresh KA. Overview of the American Heart Association "Get with the Guidelines" programs: coronary heart disease, stroke, and heart failure. *Crit Pathw Cardiol.* 2006;5(4):179-186.
2. American Heart Association. The Guideline Advantage. 2011. http://www.guidelineadvantage.org/TGA/. Accessed May 7, 2012.
3. National Cardiovascular Disease Registry. NCDR® ACTION Registry®-GWTG™ Home Page. http://www.ncdr.com/WebNCDR/Action/default.aspx. Accessed April 23, 2012.
4. American College of Cardiology. NCDR®. 2011. http://www.ncdr.com/webncdr/common/. Accessed May 7, 2012.
5. Hoekstra JW, et al. Improving the care of patients with non-ST-elevation acute coronary syndromes in the emergency department: the CRUSADE initiative. *Acad Emerg Med.* 2002;9(11):1146-1155.

6. Society of Thoracic Surgeons. STS National Database | STS. http://sts.org/national-database. Accessed May 7, 2012.

7. Fonarow GC. The Acute Decompensated Heart Failure National Registry (ADHERE): opportunities to improve care of patients hospitalized with acute decompensated heart failure. *Rev Cardiovasc Med.* 2003;4 (suppl) 7:S21-30.

8. Outcome Sciences, Inc. OPTIMIZE-HF home page. 2005. http://optimize-hf.org/. Accessed May 7, 2012.

9. Spertus JA, et al. The Prospective Registry Evaluating Myocardial Infarction: Events and Recovery (PREMIER)—evaluating the impact of myocardial infarction on patient outcomes. *Am Heart J.* 2006;151(3):589-597.

10. Arnold SV, et al. Translational Research Investigating Underlying Disparities in Acute Myocardial Infarction Patients' Health Status (TRIUMPH): design and rationale of a prospective multicenter registry. *Circ Cardiovasc Qual Outcomes.* 2011;4(4):467-476.

11. Centers for Medicare & Medicaid Services. Medicare Enrollment Reports. http://www.cms.gov/Research-Statistics-Data-and-Systems/Statistics-Trends-and-Reports/MedicareEnrpts/index.html. Accessed May 7, 2012.

12. Centers for Medicare & Medicaid Services. Carrier Line Items. 2012. https://www.cms.gov/Research-Statistics-Data-and-Systems/Statistics-Trends-and-Reports/BSAPUFS/Carrier_Line_Items.html. Accessed May 7, 2012.

13. Centers for Medicare & Medicaid Services. Denominator LDS. 2012. https://www.cms.gov/Research-Statistics-Data-and-Systems/Files-for-Order/LimitedDataSets/DenominatorLDS.html. Accessed May 7, 2012.

14. Centers for Medicare & Medicaid Services. Medicare Provider Analysis and Review File. 2012. https://www.cms.gov/Research-Statistics-Data-and-Systems/Files-for-Order/IdentifiableDataFiles/MedicareProviderAnalysisandReviewFile.html. Accessed May 7, 2012.

15. Centers for Medicare & Medicaid Services. Medicare Current Beneficiary Survey (MCBS). 2012. http://www.cms.gov/Research-Statistics-Data-and-Systems/Research/ MCBS/index.html?redirect=/mcbs. Accessed May 7, 2012.

16. Centers for Medicare & Medicaid Services. MAX General Information. 2012. https://www.cms.gov/Research-Statistics-Data-and-Systems/Computer-Data-and-Systems/MedicaidDataSourcesGenInfo/MAX GeneralInformation.html. Accessed May 7, 2012.

17. US Department of Veterans Affairs. VHA Medical SAS® Datasets—Description. http://www.virec.research.va.gov/DataSourcesName/Medical-SAS-Datasets/SAS.htm. Accessed May 7, 2012.

18. US Department of Veterans Affairs. Pharmacy Benefits Management Services (PBM)—Database. http://www.virec.research.va.gov/DataSourcesName/PBM/PBM.htm. Accessed May 7, 2012.

19. US Department of Veterans Affairs. VHA Decision Support System (DSS)—Introduction. http://www.virec.research.va.gov/DataSourcesName/DSS/DSSintro.htm. Accessed May 7, 2012.

20. US Department of Veterans Affairs. VHA Vital Status File. http://www.virec. research.va.gov/DataSourcesName/VitalStatus/VitalStatus.htm. Accessed May 7, 2012.
21. Agency for Healthcare Research and Quality. Health Care: Healthcare Cost and Utilization Project (HCUP) Subdirectory Page. http://www.ahrq.gov/ data/hcup/. Accessed May 7, 2012.
22. Agency for Healthcare Research and Quality. Medical Expenditure Panel Survey Home. http://meps.ahrq.gov/mepsweb/. Accessed May 7, 2012.
23. Cecil G. Sheps Center for Health Services Research, University of North Carolina at Chapel Hill. MarketScan® Commercial Claims and Encounters and Medicare Supplemental Databases. 2012. http://www.shepscenter.unc. edu/marketscan/index.html. Accessed May 7, 2012.
24. Division of Research, Kaiser Permanente. Research Topics. http://www.dor. kaiser.org/external/DORExternal/research/index.aspx. Accessed May 7, 2012.
25. Quan H, Parsons GA, Ghali WA. Validity of information on comorbidity derived from ICD-9-CCM administrative data. *Med Care.* 2002;40(8):675-685.
26. Hammill BG, et al. Linking inpatient clinical registry data to Medicare claims data using indirect identifiers. *Am Heart J.* 2009;157(6):995-1000.
27. Méray N, Reitsma JB, Ravelli ACJ, Bonsel GJ. Probabilistic record linkage is a valid and transparent tool to combine databases without a patient identification number. *J Clin Epidemiol.* 2007;60(9):883-891.

CHAPTER TWELVE

Observational Study Designs

Bradley G. Hammill

INTRODUCTION

Observational studies in clinical research can be classified as either analytic or descriptive (Table 12–1). Analytic observational studies are similar to randomized, controlled clinical trials in that the goal is to estimate the causal effect of an exposure on an outcome. Also similar to trials, analytic observational studies always include some type of comparison group, against which the experience of the exposed group is compared. Well-designed analytic studies can generate strong evidence for or against a stated hypothesis. Descriptive studies, on the other hand, aim to describe the characteristics or experiences of a particular patient group. Even well-designed descriptive studies cannot be used to draw strong conclusions about the effect of an exposure on an outcome. Instead, these studies are often used to generate study questions that can then be tested by more rigorous methods.

Although many observational study designs are available to researchers (1), a few are most widely used and will be described below. The analytic study designs presented are the case-control study and the cohort study. The descriptive study designs presented are the ecologic study, the cross-sectional prevalence survey, and case reports or case series.

ANALYTIC STUDY DESIGNS

Case-Control Studies

In a case-control study, the study population is selected based on a person's outcome status (2). For most case-control studies, the outcome is

TABLE 12–1

Comparison of features of analytic and descriptive study designs

	Analytic designs		Descriptive designs		
	Case-control study	Cohort study	Prevalence study	Ecologic study	Case report/ case series
Study purpose	Hypothesis testing	Hypothesis testing	Hypothesis generating	Hypothesis generating	Hypothesis generating
Primary study characteristics	Selection of study population by outcome status Need to ascertain prior exposures	Selection of study population by exposure status Need to ascertain subsequent outcomes	Single point-in-time survey of exposures and outcomes	Exposure and outcome data are aggregate measures	Detailed information regarding one or multiple interesting medical cases
Typical study population size	Small	Large	Can be small or large	(Not person level)	Very small
Temporal relationship between exposure and outcome	Difficult to establish	Easier to establish	Unknown	Difficult to establish	Usually established

Best use of study design	When outcome is rare	When exposure is rare	To establish prevalence of a disease in the sampled population	When it is infeasible to measure exposure at the individual level (e.g., environmental exposures)	To report initial results or potential safety signals for a new therapy or procedure
Primary challenge	Selection of appropriate controls. Avoiding differential recall bias when assessing exposure	For prospective designs, following study participants over time and waiting for events to occur	Not usually possible to discern timing of exposures and outcomes	No assurance that exposed persons are the same as those who experienced the outcome	No control group for comparison. Very limited population size

a disease. Cases are those that have or have had the outcome. Controls are those that lack the outcome. Cases are usually identified when they initially seek treatment for the condition of interest. Health system databases and disease-specific registries can be helpful for identifying cases. Controls are identified in any number of ways, including selecting them at random from the population or from within the same health-care delivery system or geographic area as the cases. The principle that guides the selection of controls is that they must be representative of the underlying population that generated the cases. At a minimum, this means the controls must have been eligible to have had the outcome of interest. Once the cases and controls have been selected, the prior exposure status of each study member is ascertained; then, statistical analysis is used to determine whether or not the exposure rates differ between the case group and the control group.

There are multiple advantages of this design. Most case-control studies are modestly sized and can be completed relatively quickly. Because there is no need to wait for events to occur, the major time costs incurred are those related to identifying controls and interviewing selected cases and controls about their exposure status. The case-control study design is also well suited to the study of rare outcomes. Rare types of cancer, for example, may be difficult to observe in any given cohort, but a registry of patients who developed that cancer might be a suitable starting point for a case-control study.

The challenges of the case-control design should not be overlooked, however. First, identifying a representative sample of controls can be difficult and expensive. A more convenient control group might be available, but its exposure rate might not reflect the baseline rate in the population that generated the cases. Second, asking study participants to recall details about past exposure can be problematic, especially if the exposure was not recent. This introduces the possibility of differential recall, if cases have given more thought about their potential exposures than controls have.

An example of a case-control study in the cardiology literature comes from Christiansen et al., who examined whether glucocorticoid use was associated with incident atrial fibrillation (3). Their cases, selected from hospital records, were patients who had had an inpatient diagnosis of incident atrial fibrillation. Controls were matched for age and sex. With more than 20,000 cases and 200,000 controls, this large case-control study was made possible through the use of population-based medical care databases in Denmark. Exposure to glucocorticoids was ascertained by searching pharmacy databases. Because these pharmacy data already existed for both cases and controls, this study could avoid some of the ascertainment bias present in typical epidemiological case-control studies that rely on self-reports of prior exposures. In the end, the authors found that the risk of atrial fibrillation nearly doubled with the use of glucocorticoids.

Cohort Studies

Unlike a case-control study, a cohort study begins by classifying exposure status among a group at risk for having the outcome (4). In some cohort studies, the actual selection of study participants is based on exposure status. This is especially important if the exposure of interest is rare. Only after exposure status has been determined does event ascertainment occur. Events can be ascertained either prospectively or retrospectively, but in both situations the outcome must follow the exposure. In a prospective cohort study, both the exposed group and the unexposed (or comparison) group are followed over time as events occur. In a retrospective cohort study, longitudinal data will have already been collected for the study group, meaning the events will have already occurred and simply must be tallied. Statistical analysis for a cohort study determines whether or not the outcome rates differ between the exposed group and the comparison group.

Well-designed cohort studies have some important characteristics. First, the relative timing of the exposure and the outcome is more certain in a cohort study than in a case-control study. Second, ascertainment of the exposure should be unbiased because the outcome has not yet occurred when the exposure is measured. Third, ascertainment of the outcome should also be unbiased if procedures are in place to collect events systematically for all study subjects, regardless of exposure status.

If cohort data have already been collected, a retrospective cohort study can be completed inexpensively and quickly. On the other hand, a prospective cohort study can be expensive and take years to complete. Following study participants over time is hampered if they move away; it is impossible if they opt out of the study. Retrospective cohort studies also can be limited, if necessary exposure or outcome information was not collected during the initial encounters. There is little ability to go back and obtain additional historical data.

The National Heart, Lung, and Blood Institute has funded a number of prospective cohort studies of the development of cardiovascular and related diseases in the United States. The Multi-Ethnic Study of Atherosclerosis (MESA) is one such study. Nearly 7,000 adults from 6 communities were enrolled between 2000 and 2002. Periodic follow-up examinations have been performed since the inception of the cohort. One example publication based on MESA data is by Kestenbaum et al. (5). They examined whether differences in kidney function were associated with incident hypertension in patients who lacked hypertension at baseline. Their exposure of interest, kidney function, was measured using cystatin C levels during the first data collection period. The development of hypertension was determined in subsequent examinations, ensuring that the timings of exposure and outcome were appropriate. The average follow-up in the cohort was just over 3 years. They found that higher levels of cystatin C were significantly associated with an increased risk of incident hypertension. Because this was a prospective cohort, the investigators had to wait for follow-up examinations before they could determine whether any incident disease had developed.

DESCRIPTIVE STUDY DESIGNS (4)

Ecologic Studies

Ecologic studies are those in which measurement is performed at the population level rather than at the individual level, but for which the study hypothesis involves individual-level exposures and outcomes (6,7). An ecologic study can compare outcome rates between populations in different geographic regions that have different exposure levels, or it can examine outcomes rates within a single population over time to see how they correlate with changes in exposure levels over time. One main reason that researchers use this design is that aggregated rates of disease and other population characteristics are often readily available and can be analyzed quickly and inexpensively. Conclusions from these studies are weaker than conclusions based on other designs, however, because there is no way to ensure that the exposed members of a population were the same ones who had the outcomes contributing to the observed rates. Without this information, ecologic studies are primarily used for evidence generation.

One representative ecologic study examined the effect of air pollution on cardiovascular-related hospital admissions (8). Using data from the Environmental Protection Agency, Schwartz obtained daily measurements of air pollution for eight counties around the United States. Specific air pollution measures included the quantities of small particulate matter and of carbon monoxide in the air. The outcome of interest was the number of daily hospital admissions for cardiovascular causes in the same counties. Increases in small particulate matter and carbon monoxide levels were significantly associated with small increases in number of admissions. Of note, this study relied on county-level data and could not measure both outcome and exposure at the individual level. Indeed, individual-level measurement of air pollution and other environmental exposures is extremely difficult. As a result, the study of health risks due to environmental exposures is one area of research that relies heavily on ecologic studies.

Cross-Sectional (Prevalence) Studies

Cross-sectional studies collect data about health and exposure status of a population at a single point in time. Unlike cohort studies, members of a cross-sectional study are not followed longitudinally. So although it is possible to compare exposure rates among surveyed individuals with and without a disease, it is not possible to draw conclusions about causation because the timing of the collected information is difficult or impossible to determine. In fact, because of the lack of information about timing, these are often called *prevalence studies.*

The best cross-sectional studies use statistical sampling to select study individuals who accurately represent the population of interest. This, in turn, makes any study results readily generalizable. For example, estimates of the prevalence of disease and the prevalence of exposures in the surveyed population will be accurate measures of population prevalence. For this reason, cross-sectional studies are useful for estimating the disease burden in a population, which can be useful for healthcare planning. As with other descriptive designs, they are also useful for reporting interesting exposure–outcome associations that might merit further investigation.

The National Health and Nutrition Examination Survey (NHANES) is an ongoing cross-sectional survey used to assess the health of adult Americans. It employs a complex sampling design to ensure that the selected respondents are representative of the national population. Selvin and Erlinger used data from the 1999 to 2000 NHANES to examine the prevalence of and risk factors for peripheral arterial disease (PAD) (9). They found that just over 4% of the US adult population had PAD. This finding was important in and of itself, given that previous estimates of PAD prevalence had ranged from 3% to 30%. They went on to report that PAD was positively associated with many other health conditions, including diabetes, reduced kidney function, and hypercholesterolemia. They were careful not to infer causation between PAD and any other condition, precisely because determination of causality is difficult in a prevalence study. For example, they pointed out that higher levels of C-reactive protein, a marker of inflammation, in people with PAD could be either a cause or an effect of the disease.

Case Reports and Case Series

A case report is a written presentation of a particular medical case encountered by a physician. A case series is an aggregation of case reports. Case reports and case series are most useful when a clustering of cases share some unusual feature. This clustering could be geographic or it could represent patients who share a specific characteristic or treatment. The unusual feature can be a rare or previously unrecognized disease, a previously unreported association, or a novel therapy. Many published case series are the first indication that a rare adverse event might be associated with a therapy or procedure. Because clinical trials are not usually powered to detected rare events, case series can perform an important function in detection of safety signals. More formal testing would need to follow to confirm suspected associations. Toward this end, the identified cases could be used in a subsequent case-control study.

Gaita et al. presented one of the first case series for radio frequency catheter ablation of atrial fibrillation in 1998 (10). They were interested in finding out whether ablation in the right atrium was a safe and effective procedure for atrial fibrillation. Their study population included 16 consecutive patients with idiopathic atrial fibrillation for whom drug therapy had failed. After about a year of follow-up, 9 of these patients (56%) had no recurrence of atrial fibrillation and were considered successfully ablated. Additionally, they observed no complications during the ablation procedure in their study population. Typical of published case reports and case series, the findings are suggestive; in this case, that ablation for atrial fibrillation is safe and effective. However, without a control group, it is not possible to know what proportion of similar cases of atrial fibrillation might have resolved on their own over the same period. And without a large sample, it is difficult to know if there truly are any safety problems. Adverse events that occur at a rate of even 1 per 100 require a study population many times larger than the one presented.

CONCLUSIONS

Each of the study designs described in this chapter represents a different approach to answering a research question. If possible, researchers should strive to conduct a well-designed analytic study, which should lead to a stronger conclusion than any descriptive study. In the end, of course, that may not be possible. The selection of one design over another depends on both the details of the study question (patient population, exposure, and outcome) and the resources available to carry out the study (time, money, and existing data sources).

REFERENCES

1. Rothman KJ, Greenland S, Lash TL. *Modern Epidemiology*. 3rd ed. Philadelphia, PA: Lippincott, Williams & Wilkins; 2008.
2. Wacholder S. Design issues in case-control studies. *Stat Methods Med Res*. 1995;4(4):293-309.
3. Christiansen CF, et al. Glucocorticoid use and risk of atrial fibrillation or flutter: a population-based, case-control study. *Arch Intern Med*. 2009;169 (18):1677-1683.
4. Prentice RL. Design issues in cohort studies. *Stat Methods Med Res*. 1995;4 (4):273-292.
5. Kestenbaum B, et al. Differences in kidney function and incident hypertension: the multi-ethnic study of atherosclerosis. *Ann Intern Med*. 2008;148(7): 501-508.
6. Tu JV, Ko DT. Ecological studies and cardiovascular outcomes research. *Circulation*. 2008;118(24):2588-2593.
7. Morgenstern H. Ecologic studies in epidemiology: concepts, principles, and methods. *Annu Rev Public Health*. 1995;16:61-81.
8. Schwartz J. Air pollution and hospital admissions for heart disease in eight U.S. counties. *Epidemiology*. 1999;10(1):17-22.
9. Selvin E, Erlinger TP. Prevalence of and risk factors for peripheral arterial disease in the United States: results from the National Health and Nutrition Examination Survey, 1999-2000. *Circulation*. 2004;110(6):738-743.
10. Gaita F, et al. Atrial mapping and radiofrequency catheter ablation in patients with idiopathic atrial fibrillation. Electrophysiological findings and ablation results. *Circulation*. 1998;97(21):2136-2145.

CHAPTER THIRTEEN

Challenges of Observational Designs

David M. Vock

INTRODUCTION

Although randomized controlled experiments remain the gold standard for medical research, observational studies—studies in which the researcher does not assign or alter any factor of interest—still play an important role.

Some research questions lend themselves exclusively to observational designs. In many instances, the factor of interest cannot be controlled by the investigator. Consider a study on the impact of race on the effectiveness of pegylated interferon and ribavirin in treating chronic hepatitis C virus infection (1). The researcher cannot randomly assign being Caucasian to one group of patients and being African American to another group; such a study must be observational. Similarly, genome-wide association studies must be observational because researchers cannot alter people's genetic makeup. Other research questions might not involve relating a factor of interest to an outcome. Studies that seek only to characterize an outcome in a single population of interest will, by definition, be observational. For example, a recent study sought to determine the proportion of patients who lost independence or physical function 1 year after suffering a myocardial infarction (MI) (2).

Even for research questions that could be answered by a randomized trial, an observational study might be advantageous. Randomized trials are costly and time-consuming to run and entail navigating and complying with complex regulations (see references 3 and 4 for examples). Using data from a registry or a previously completed trial investigating a different research question would allow analysis of data far more quickly. In fact, more data might be available from registries than could be obtained in a new trial. For example, consider early studies on the efficacy of coronary artery bypass grafting (CABG) compared with percutaneous coronary intervention (PCI). A pooled analysis of eight randomized controlled trials involved a total of only 3,371 patients (an average 421 patients per trial) (5), whereas an analysis of a single registry included 6,814 patients (6). Observational data also can allow researchers to consider a wider group of patients than would be possible in a controlled trial; many randomized experiments exclude large subpopulations, particularly those that have other comorbidities or significant risk factors. Finally, in many instances, it can be unethical to consider randomizing some factors that are known to compromise patient health, such as smoking status or physical activity level.

Although using observational data for biomedical research can have advantages over implementing and running a randomized controlled trial, there are many pitfalls in using observational data that can undermine the validity of conclusions drawn from such analysis. Investigators must be aware of these potential problems so that they can be mitigated when possible and acknowledged as limitations otherwise.

This chapter focuses on scenarios in which the data have not been collected to specifically answer the question of interest—that is, when general registry data or data from a previous trial are used. (Observational studies in which the investigator designs the data collection to answer a question that lends itself exclusively to an observational design are less prone to the pitfalls we will discuss, although certainly not immune.) The chapter refers to the factor being studied relative to an outcome as "treatment," even if the factor has nothing to do with medical therapy and cannot be assigned by the investigator.

Many types of named biases and issues can arise from using observational data (Table 13–1). We discuss those most commonly encountered in

TABLE 13–1
Types of bias

Nonresponse bias	Information bias
Withdrawal bias	Recall bias
Volunteer bias	Response bias
Selection bias (convenience sample)	Survivor bias/healthy worker bias

biomedical research, but the underlying cause of most biases is either confounding or obtaining a sample that is not representative of the population of interest. In fact, the underlying problem with confounding, as we will discuss shortly, is that we do not obtain a representative sample of the population of interest in all treatment groups. Therefore, if we can recognize situations where the sample is not representative of the population of interest, we can recognize almost all problems associated with observational data and are free from having to memorize a long list of pitfalls. This highlights the importance of clearly defining the population.

KEY CONCEPTS

As a motivating example, we consider the research question in the report by Pocock et al. (5). The investigators were interested in determining the difference in the average survival time after CABG compared with PCI among American adults with coronary artery disease (CAD) who have just undergone coronary catheterization. In this example, the *population*, or group of patients the investigator is interested in studying, is all US adults with CAD who had an indication for and underwent coronary catheterization. The *parameter* of interest, or summary measure of the population, is the difference between the mean survival time *if the entire population had undergone CABG* and the mean survival time *if the entire population had undergone PCI*. Because it is not logistically feasible to collect survival times on all US patients with CAD, nor is it possible to have patients undergo both CABG and PCI simultaneously, we must collect data on smaller numbers of patients who undergo only one of the procedures. In other words, we obtain data from a *sample* of all patients included in the population. Assuming for now that all patients were followed until death, we can calculate the difference in the average survival time for CABG versus PCI among the patients included in our sample. A summary measure of the sample, such as the difference in average survival time, is called a *statistic*. We hope to use the computed statistics to *infer* likely values for the parameter.

The difference in the mean survival time calculated in our sample is not likely to equal the true mean difference in the population, although we hope that the two would be close. Some of the difference may result from *sampling error*, perhaps more accurately described as *sampling variability* or *sampling deviation*. If we redid the study using the same methods to identify and select subjects, we would obtain a different sample and, thus, a different statistic. The difference between the two statistics calculated from the two samples results from sampling variability. This deviation occurs because we observe data only on a portion of the total population. We might consider taking samples from the population and calculating the statistic of interest many times, with the hope that the average of the statistics calculated from each sample would equal the parameter. If this is the case, then the statistic is considered a *valid* estimate of the parameter. We can ensure that the sample statistic is valid by guaranteeing that the sample is representative of the population. Any discrepancy between the average of the statistic and the parameter results from *systemic error*, and the discrepancy is known as *bias*. This chapter identifies scenarios where the sample is not likely to be representative of the population

Confounding

A *confounder* is any variable associated with both the outcome of interest and the likelihood of receiving a particular treatment in the sample selected by the researcher. In other words, a confounder is any prognostic factor (i.e., a factor associated with outcome) that is also used to decide what treatment a patient received. Continuing the previous example (5), the data used in the analysis were obtained from a registry of patients at an academic medical center. The researchers did not decide which treatment the patient received (CABG or PCI); this was left to the patients and physicians. Although the cardiologists presumably followed clinical guidelines, at the time of the analysis there was little consensus on the preferred therapy and there was significant variability in which treatment patients received. However, patients undergoing CABG tended to have more diseased vessels than those undergoing PCI. If the researchers had simply computed the average survival time in patients undergoing each procedure, they could not have determined whether differences in survival reflected differences in treatment or differences in the average number of diseased vessels. The number of diseased vessels is thus a confounder for the effect of treatment on survival (Figure 13–1). The difference in the average survival time observed in the sample will be biased for the difference in the survival time in the population of interest because patients who underwent CABG in our sample tended to have more diseased vessels than the average person in the population, whereas those undergoing PCI had, on average, fewer diseased vessels than observed in the population. In short, the sample of patients in each treatment arm is not representative of the entire population of interest.

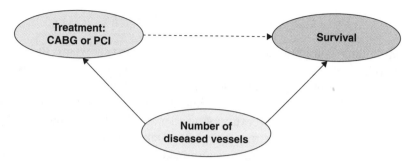

FIGURE 13–1. Illustration of confounding. The number of diseased vessels influences the likelihood of a patient receiving CABG versus PCI in Pocock et al. (5). Because patients who have multiple diseased vessels tend to have shorter survival times, the number of diseased vessels is a confounder. If investigators simply compute the average survival time among patients receiving CABG or PCI, they cannot determine whether a difference in survival reflects differences in treatment or differences in the average number of diseased vessels.

We again emphasize the importance of defining the population of interest. Consider a similar scenario as given above, except that now we are interested in determining the difference in survival time between patients who undergo CABG and patients who undergo PCI. Here we are not concerned with the difference in treatment among *all* patients with CAD who have just undergone coronary catheterization. Rather, we want to examine the difference in outcome among all US patients with CAD who *received* CABG or PCI. In this case, our samples will be representative of the populations of interest and there is no confounding. In other words, by redefining or restricting the population of interest, we can eliminate confounding.

Confounding and Randomized Trials

Randomized trials are considered the gold standard of clinical research because they avoid issues of confounding by randomly assigning treatment. There are no factors that are associated with treatment assignment and outcome, and patients assigned to each treatment will be representative of the population from which patients were identified for recruitment. In other words, so long as we have recruited patients who are representative of the population of interest, patients in each treatment arm will be representative of the population if we randomly assign treatment.

Time-Dependent Confounding

Confounding is traditionally described using scenarios where the treatment is allocated at a fixed point in time (e.g., immediately after catheterization) and might be associated with other prognostic factors measured at that time point. However, confounding also occurs in studies in which treatment decisions vary over time. Consider the situation encountered by Pieper et al. (7), in which the aspirin dose taken by patients with acute coronary syndromes (ACS) was determined by the patient and attending physician and allowed to change over time in response to changes in clinical status. Investigators might be interested in determining the effect of aspirin dose on future MI. Because the aspirin dose was nonrandomized, the aspirin regimen that patients followed was not controlled by the investigator— physicians were free to change the dose at any time. One method of addressing the research question would be to examine the rates of MI among those taking similar average doses of aspirin over time, but aspirin use can be confounded by other prognostic factors that might vary over time. For example, an increase in blood pressure might be an indication for starting aspirin. In this example, the confounder is time dependent; it is the current blood pressure, not the blood pressure upon entry into the study that is associated with starting aspirin.

Even within randomized trials, secondary subgroup analyses can be observational. Time-dependent confounding is crucial to understanding the dangers of examining treatment effects in subgroups that are defined by *postrandomization covariates*, that is, covariates that are measured or defined after the study drug has been randomized. A question that has arisen from trials of platelet glycoprotein (GP) IIb/IIIa inhibitors in non-ST-elevation ACS is whether the treatment effect differs in patients undergoing PCI compared with receiving medical therapy alone (7). In these trials, treatment is randomized at enrollment, so there are no concerns about confounding when analyzing the effect of GP IIb/IIIa inhibitors compared with placebo on average survival time after enrollment. However, the investigators are also interested in assessing the average difference in survival time between those taking GP IIb/IIIa inhibitors and those taking placebo among patients who eventually undergo PCI. The population of interest is now everyone who eventually underwent PCI. Note that treatment assignment was not randomized in this population, nor would it be feasible to randomize treatment at baseline among the subgroup that eventually underwent PCI. In fact, the randomized treatment assignment might affect the likelihood of undergoing PCI; Pieper et al. (7) describe several biologically possible reasons why the likelihood of undergoing PCI might differ between the active treatment and control arms. Thus, the average patient given GP IIb/IIIa inhibitors and undergoing PCI might be prognostically different from the average patient given placebo and undergoing PCI. After PCI, the two initially randomized treatment groups represent two different populations. Here, treatment history is the confounder.

Another example of comparing postrandomization subgroups is when investigators compare the effects of randomized therapy (that was randomized at hospital admission, say) among all patients who were discharged within 30 days of hospital admission. As before, the subgroup of interest, patients discharged within 30 days of admission, is determined after treatment randomization. Estimates of the effect of therapy in this subgroup are not representative of the effect of therapy in all patients who are hospitalized, because treatment history may be a confounder. The bias in the estimate of treatment efficacy is often referred to as *survivor bias*, because we are examining effects only among survivors, patients who were discharged within 30 days. In epidemiological studies of the effect of toxic exposure, this bias is referred to as the *healthy worker bias*; frequently we sample only from workers who remain (survive) in the workforce even though we are interested in the effects of all people who were exposed.

Besides randomly assigning treatment or redefining the population of interest, bias that results from confounding can in some instances be overcome by using sophisticated statistical methods and usually strong assumptions (see Chapter 15). However, we must know and have measured all confounders for these methods to yield valid results. Unfortunately there is no way to determine whether all confounders have been measured. When possible, it is best to try to avoid situations when confounding is likely to be present.

NONREPRESENTATIVE SAMPLE

When a nonrepresentative sample is used, results can be biased. The reason bias arises depends on whether two or more treatments are being compared or whether an outcome is being described for a single population (e.g., prevalence of disease). In the first case, bias results when the treatment difference among excluded or underrepresented subgroups is not the same as the treatment difference in other subgroups. In the latter case, bias occurs when an excluded or underrepresented subgroup has a different prevalence of the disease in question. This is important to understand because medical researchers can rarely obtain samples that are representative of the population in all facets imaginable. For purely illustrative purposes, consider a study that randomly samples all patients with diabetes mellitus but excludes patients born on the tenth day of each month. Because we are interested in all patients who have diabetes mellitus, technically this sample is nonrepresentative, but the day of the month on which a patient was born is unlikely to relate to the prevalence of the disease.

Nonresponse Bias

Nonresponse bias occurs when subjects identified by the investigator for inclusion in the study fail to provide data for or participate in the study, and the patients who do not enroll are clinically different than those who do. For example, patients enrolled in trials or registries that have long-term commitments often miss follow-up visits or might withdraw from the study completely. Patients with all data collected might not be representative of the patients with missing data because patients who withdraw from the study or miss intermediate follow-up visits are often not improving on their assigned therapy or are having severe side effects. The bias that results from subjects leaving a study is frequently referred to as *withdrawal bias*. Patients identified for inclusion in a study but who do not consent to enroll in a trial or registry can be considered another form of nonresponse. This nonresponse can lead to bias because patients who do enroll and assume the risks of a clinical trial are unlikely to represent the entire population of interest. In other words, there may be some bias, often referred to as *volunteer bias*, because the patients who *self-select* into the study are not representative.

Selection Bias

Whereas nonresponse bias reflects a sample becoming less representative by patients refusing to supply data once enrolled in the study, selection bias reflects a researcher selecting a nonrepresentative population of interest from the outset. This often happens in observational studies when the sample comes from a completed trial with strict inclusion/exclusion criteria but the researcher is interested in studying a much larger cross section of patients. Both registries and clinical trials often have data only from small networks of clinics and hospitals. Patients included in these networks might not be representative of all patients across the country with a particular disease, and the sample selected is referred to as a *convenience sample*.

Information Bias

Even if we identify a sample and those patients are representative of the broader population of interest, we may not obtain information that is representative of the broader population. For self-reported measures, patients may systematically not provide truthful information (knowingly or unknowingly) so that the data obtained are not representative. Self-reported measures are commonly used in registries and some trials where follow-up information is obtained from telephone interviews. Patients may not be able to recall treatments received or medical events especially if the interviews are scheduled far apart. The bias that results from the fact that patients sometimes cannot remember medical history is known as *recall bias*. In addition, patients may try to respond in ways that are more socially acceptable or that they perceive as being beneficial for medical research. For example, patients may be more likely to deceive the researcher that they are continuing on study medication when in fact they are not than the converse. The tendency of subjects to supply answers that are considered more socially acceptable can lead to biased parameter estimates and is known as *response bias*.

As with confounding, if we know *how* the sample is not representative, we can use statistical methods that allow us to obtain a valid estimate for the population of interest. This usually requires making some strict assumptions, however. It is best to try to obtain a representative sample.

CONCLUSIONS

Observational studies remain an important part of biomedical research. As discussed at length in the introduction, observational studies are cheaper, quicker, and less burdensome than experimental research and may be able to test certain hypotheses over a broader population than experimental research can. However, there are several potential problems with observational data that may prevent researchers from drawing valid conclusions. Most notably, the effect of treatment may be confounded with other covariates, and the sample from which data are collected may not be representative of the broader population of interest. A common theme that will be discussed in subsequent chapters is that if we know the potential confounders and how the sample may not be representative, then statistical methods exist that allow us to obtain valid inferences from the population. The existence of advanced statistical methods does not obviate the need to understand these problems, however. Indeed, we can never be certain that we have enumerated all confounders or all ways in which a sample is not representative. Furthermore, no statistical test can evaluate whether all cofounders have been identified. Good observational analyses always explicitly state these potential limitations.

REFERENCES

1. Conjeevaram HS, et al. Peginterferon and ribavirin treatment in African American and Caucasian American patients with hepatitis C genotype 1. *Gastroenterology.* 2006;131(2):470-477.
2. Dodson JA, et al. Physical function and independence 1 year after myocardial infarction: observations from the Translational Research Investigating Underlying disparities in recovery from acute Myocardial infarction: Patients' Health status registry. *Am Heart J.* 2012;163(5):790-796.
3. Glickman SW, et al. Ethical and scientific implications of the globalization of clinical research. *N Engl J Med.* 2009;360(8):816-823.
4. Califf RM. Simple principles of clinical trials remain powerful. *JAMA.* 2005; 293(4):489-491.
5. Pocock SJ, et al. Meta-analysis of randomised trials comparing coronary angioplasty with bypass surgery. *Lancet.* 1995;346(8984):1184-1189.
6. Jones RH, et al. Long-term survival benefits of coronary artery bypass grafting and percutaneous transluminal angioplasty in patients with coronary artery disease. *J Thorac Cardiovasc Surg.* 1996;111(5):1013-1025.
7. Pieper KS, et al. Differential treatment benefit of platelet glycoprotein IIb/IIIa inhibition with percutaneous coronary intervention versus medical therapy for acute coronary syndromes: exploration of methods. *Circulation.* 2004; 109(5):641-646.

CHAPTER FOURTEEN

Specific Regression Techniques

Phillip J. Schulte and Laine E. Thomas

INTRODUCTION

$\mathbf{R}$egression is a tool used by statisticians and clinicians to establish or identify a relationship between one or more explanatory covariates and a response variable (outcome). Many textbooks are devoted to specific regression models and strategies. In particular, *Regression Modeling Strategies with Applications to Linear Models, Logistic Regression and Survival Analysis* by Harrell (1) is an excellent reference. In this chapter, we briefly summarize and exemplify the techniques that are fundamental to outcomes research.

First we address common, or "macro," issues in regression modeling, regardless of the scale of outcome. We discuss the purpose of an analysis and the relationship to covariate selection, model complexity, and criteria for model performance. Focus is placed on interpretation of models on a "macro" scale. We then focus on features of specific models (linear, logistic, and hazards regression), paying particular attention to the hypotheses and data behind an analysis. Parameters and output are interpreted on a "micro" scale for each of the three regression methods.

GENERAL STRATEGIES

Purpose

Before building a regression model, the statistician and clinician should discuss the modeling purpose, key hypotheses, and available data. Each of these will guide an appropriate regression analysis.

189

The purpose of an analysis may not be straightforward or singular. Some common purposes seen in practice are to establish a predictive model for an outcome (prediction), identify covariate associations that can inform understanding of disease etiology (association), or examine a specific variable of interest while adjusting for the effects of others (adjustment). If we knew the "true model," including all important variables and their functional relationships with outcome, then model would be useful for all purposes. In practice, we do not know the truth, and our decisions have trade-offs. Understanding the purpose of the model helps us create a model that is useful, albeit imperfect.As its name suggests, a predictive model is used when clinicians are interested in predicting the outcome for future patients based on currently available data. Having a predicted risk of outcome can guide treatment and therapies as well as inform the patient. The goal is to achieve precise predictions of future outcomes, rather than interpreting specific parameter estimates. There is no benefit from including covariates for which the effect cannot be well estimated. Researchers might be willing to yield some bias in individual covariate estimates in exchange for greater precision. Hence, statisticians and clinicians must work to identify the covariates that are the most important to predicting outcome. Automated variable-selection techniques are commonly employed; such techniques are discussed below. However, any variable selection should still be guided, in part, by clinical practice. In a predictive study, interpretation of the model can be largely focused on performance statistics, such as the C-index, to evaluate the model prediction as a whole. Some of these predictive assessment tools are described below. Researchers often publish an entire predictive model or design a nomogram to aid practitioners in establishing patient risk using a predictive model (1).

Roe et al. (2) exemplify the dual purpose of studying association but emphasizing prediction. In this case, the outcome was long-term mortality in older patients with non-ST-segment elevation myocardial infarction (MI) enrolled in the Can Rapid risk stratification of Unstable angina patients Suppress ADverse outcomes with Early implementation of the ACC/AHA guidelines? (CRUSADE) registry. The authors initially emphasized a comparison of associations, and relative covariate importance, in a model with 22 statistically significant variables. Subsequently, they focused on prediction, using clinical judgment to define a reduced model with 13 covariates but nearly equivalent predictive performance (comparable discrimination [C-index] 0.75 for the derivation sample of the full model versus 0.73 for the reduced model). The reduced model was slightly inferior, and does not represent an optimal strategy for prediction; however, it achieves greater simplicity and convenience with relatively little compromise in performance. The focus on prediction was further emphasized by the creation of a risk score. Of interest, they did not use an automatic variable-selection procedure but instead included all 22 univariably significant ($\alpha = 0.05$) covariates in the initial model.

Superior techniques exist for predictive modeling. However, in the very large CRUSADE registry, alternative techniques are unlikely to provide clinically different predictive performance because there is sufficient power to detect even marginally important covariates and little chance of overfitting.

At the other end of the spectrum from the prediction model is the adjustment model. Often arising when a clinician wants to examine the effect of a particular covariate, adjustment models need not employ automated variable selection. As discussed in *Chapters 13 and 15*, confounding can lead to biased coefficient estimates when the confounding variable is not properly adjusted for. Thus, in the adjustment model, focus is on minimizing the bias of the estimated coefficient by including all known confounders. Ideally, these may be identified from previous publications, including larger studies and clinically similar populations. These variables need not achieve statistical significance in the dataset being analyzed, because researchers may be willing to accept some additional "noise" to minimize bias. Overall, there is less concern for overfitting, except that excessive inappropriate covariates should not be included. For example, if a particular characteristic has been shown to be important in the literature but is not statistically significant in one's sample, it should still be adjusted for. In an adjustment study, only the particular covariate of interest must be interpreted. In fact, adjustment studies need not publish the entire model but rather mention the adjustment covariates and display output only for the covariate of interest.

For an example of an adjustment model, consider Piccini et al. (3). The authors sought to identify the relationships that two drugs for treatment of ventricular arrhythmia—amiodarone and lidocaine—had with 30-day and 6-month mortality, using data from the Global Use of Strategies To Open occluded coronary arteries in acute coronary syndromes (GUSTO)-IIb and GUSTO-III randomized controlled trials. Partly because of the secondary nature of the analysis, the authors were concerned with confounding. Thus, attempting to identify the risk attributable to each medication required adjusting for clinical characteristics. A published model for mortality in a similar population (4), along with expert guidance from the investigators, was used to identify 17 adjustment covariates. The authors noted these adjustment variables but reported hazard ratios and results only for the treatment variables of interest.

Finally, some clinicians wish to explore associations among many covariates and outcome, with a focus on the biological processes driving outcomes. This common purpose is probably the hardest to achieve. As with adjustment models, researchers want unbiased estimates because they will interpret parameters, but as with prediction, they are concerned about minimizing overfitting and want to include only important covariates. Essentially, researchers want to avoid including numerous nonsignificant covariates that would add noise to the system while complicating interpretation. Multicollinearity, when two or more variables are highly correlated and affect outcome, is a concern and thought must be given to determining the appropriate causal and biological pathway to consider. Variable-selection techniques can be employed, but a firm understanding of how covariates interact and change together should be taken into consideration during selection instead of using an "out-of-the-box" variable-selection solution that might not be very interpretable or biologically consistent. Interpretation is of the whole model, perhaps with a focus on particular biological systems of interest.

The report from Forman et al. (5) provides an example of associative modeling. (Note, however, that associative purposes vary and can be presented in many different ways.) Using data from the Heart Failure: A Controlled Trial Investigating Outcomes of exercise traiNing (HF-ACTION) study, the researchers sought an associative model for measures of exercise capacity that included age and 34 other candidate variables. The primary conclusion regarded age as a key to the pathophysiology and clinical management of reduced exercise performance in older persons with heart failure. Stepwise selection was used to select variables for their model, followed by a procedure to further isolate the most significant factors in assessing exercise capacity. Finally, for some of their models, key covariates that were considered clinically relevant were added to the models. Interactions with age were explored for each outcome. In particular, the researchers were interested in interpreting whether various covariates affecting outcomes would have differential associations with outcome at increased or decreased age values or independent of age. Estimated effects were provided for all covariates for one of the primary outcomes.

Variable-Selection Techniques

Many studies collect numerous variable measurements on subjects, some of which may be related to a particular outcome while others are not. In the presence of many candidate variables, variable selection may be employed to determine which variables to include in a final model. Traditional variable-selection techniques include forward, backward, and stepwise selection. Modern methods use penalized regression and shrinkage methods, such as the least absolute shrinkage and selection operator (LASSO) regression, adaptive LASSO, and modern variations in traditional methods, such as fast false selection rate (FSR) variable selection.

Forward, backward, and stepwise (collectively, FBS) selections are among the most common traditional variable-selection methods. They are iterative procedures that systematically introduce or remove variables from the statistical model one at a time until criteria are met.

In forward selection, researchers must specify an entry requirement, such as $P < 0.05$. Criteria can be based on a variety of statistics, such as adjusted R^2, Akaike information criterion (AIC), Bayesian information criterion (BIC), or Mallows' Cp, but commonly an F-test is employed when a corresponding P value cutoff is used. The statistical software begins by assuming there are no variables in the model. One by one, it checks a model for each variable. The variable with the smallest P value is entered into the model if it meets the entry requirement. Then the remaining variables are checked again using a model conditional on the first selected variable. Again, the smallest is selected and entered if it meets the entry criteria. This process is repeated until no more candidate variables meet the entry criteria. One consequence of this process is that the final model can contain nonsignificant variables that met the criteria for entry but do not remain significant after other variables are added.

Backward selection uses the reverse process. First, researchers must specify an exit criterion, for example, $P > 0.20$ based on a conditional F-test. The software fits a model that includes all possible candidate variables. The variable with the largest P value is selected and, if the exit criterion is satisfied, is dropped from the model. The model is then rerun without the dropped variable, and selection continues until no variable in the model meets the exit criterion.

Finally, stepwise selection employs elements of both forward and backward selection and is increasingly common in the medical literature. Both entry and exit criteria are specified. Starting with the null model, each variable is tested for entry. After a variable is entered, the model is checked for variables that meet the exit criterion. The entry–exit procedure is repeated until no remaining candidate variables meet the entry criterion and no included variables meet the exit criterion.

Some recent developments have focused on penalization or shrinkage methods. Among these modern methods, variations in LASSO regression can be applied (6). In short, LASSO estimates coefficients while optimizing model criteria such as AIC or BIC. Some coefficients are not worth estimating, because their estimates would be no better than zero according to the criteria of AIC or BIC. As a result, some estimates are set to zero while others are "shrunk" toward zero. In general, the best predictors will see very little shrinkage of estimates, whereas poor predictors will be shrunk substantially toward or even completely to zero. Variables with nonzero coefficients are interpreted as important, in the sense that they add to prediction.

Other recent developments include fast FSR variable selection (7). Fast FSR is commonly applied as an adjunct to forward selection to improve model error and decrease false selection. The procedure intentionally adds noisy, uninformative variables to the list of potential covariates and tracks them to see when they enter the model. Doing so allows the procedure to stop before allowing many poor predictors into the model, which often occurs in traditional forward selection.

No variable-selection method is without criticism. LASSO regression and adaptive LASSO are often criticized because they provide neither P values nor confidence bounds for parameter estimates. Worse is that FBS and fast FSR regression methods provide improper P values and confidence bounds. Often overlooked in medical literature, the P value provided by these traditional methods is conditional on the final model and does not account for variation induced through iterative searches and multiple comparisons made along the way. Hence, reported P values are overly optimistic; the literal use of these P values and confidence bounds might result in higher false-discovery rates, and estimates might not be validated in future studies. Such improper P values should be used only as an exploratory tool for researchers, particularly if the number of covariates tested in variable selection is large.

Biased estimates are a concern for all variable-selection methods. Under LASSO methods, all estimates are "shrunk" toward zero, some more than others. Hence, even in the most ideal scenario, LASSO estimates are biased toward zero; however, recall that for good predictors, this bias ("shrinkage") will be minimal. FBS methods can often lead to overfit models, although recent work, such as the fast FSR procedure, is starting to address this issue. If an FBS method or fast FSR identifies the true but unknown model, then the estimates would be unbiased; however, this is often unrealistic in practice.

Despite the increased use of stepwise selection in medical literature and the criticisms of each method noted above, statistical preference when developing a predictive model is typically for shrinkage methods such as LASSO and adaptive LASSO. The LASSO estimator has shown good predictive performance compared with traditional methods (8). When developing an associative model or an adjustment model, fast FSR may provide the best set of tools to minimize biased estimates while controlling for overfitting, more so than FBS methods alone. Again, any variable-selection method should not be used haphazardly, but rather guided by clinical and statistical knowledge.

Model Complexity

The study purpose also can influence other regression modeling assumptions, including model complexity. Consider two primary modeling assumptions related to linearity and interactions (additivity). First, consider whether the model will employ only linear effects or whether quadratic or linear splines should be considered. In many cases, linear effects are sufficient; but this assumption should be tested for adequacy and transformations should be made when appropriate. It is easy to show examples where a particular variable has no linear effect but a significant effect is present when splines are considered. For example, age can have a strong positive association with outcome for subjects younger than 50 but should be associated with worse/negative outcomes for those older than 50. The linear effect of age might be marginalized by the contradictory associations seen above and below the knot point.

Researchers should also decide if interactions between covariates should be considered. Interactions can quickly complicate a model that has many covariates, so interaction terms are frequently avoided unless the clinician has reason to anticipate unique subgroup associations. To illustrate complexity, suppose researchers are considering 10 covariates (age, weight, etc.) for their main effects. In this case, there are 45 possible second-order interactions (say, between age and weight), in addition to numerous higher-order interactions of 3 or more variables. Ignoring the multiple comparisons required to test the 45 interactions and refitting of the data for each would be grossly irresponsible. Thus, interactions should be considered only when expert knowledge or inquisition supports it.

When many different variables are tested and retested, multiple comparisons are being made. Without properly adjusting for the process, an overfit model can result. For example, consider 20 uncorrelated randomly distributed variables that are also completely uncorrelated with outcome. If all 20 variables were considered in a model for outcome, we would expect, by chance alone, an average of 1 of the 20 to have an observed P value <0.05. If one tests and retests many potential covariates in an unorganized and haphazard way, the probability of obtaining spurious results increases.

The big picture to consider is that trade-offs exist when making decisions regarding model complexity. Including interactions can lead to overfitting the model if no true interaction effect exists, but leaving interactions out of a model can result in some bias. Similarly, quadratic or spline terms are not always appropriate, but omission of important ones can lead to significant bias, say, by declaring age insignificant despite significant associations in certain subsets of age. At all times, one should be mindful of making multiple comparisons without proper adjustment. Again, expert opinion and biological processes should guide the use of interactions.

Roe et al. (2) exemplify these considerations. The authors evaluated the linearity of all continuous variables and used linear splines to account for nonlinearity. For example, the association between mortality and the initial hematocrit concentration was strong when hematocrit was greater than 35%, with lower hematocrit concentration corresponding to worse outcomes in this range of values, but when the hematocrit concentration was below 35%, the increment was smaller. Essentially, there was a modest plateau. Accounting for nonlinearity required additional testing for seven continuous model variables. On the other hand, there were 231 possible two-way interactions between the model covariates. Exploring all of these would have resulted in excessive multiple testing; thus these were not explored. Alternatively, a subset of biologically plausible interactions could have been explored and might have improved prediction by more accurately representing the risk of individuals who have a combination of risk factors.

Evaluation

The final general strategy discussed here concerns evaluation of models. Particularly for predictive models, it is important to evaluate model performance for predictive accuracy. Specifically, we can evaluate model discrimination, calibration, and overall performance. Discrimination is a model's predictive ability to distinguish between subjects with different responses. Calibration describes prediction bias, which is the extent of agreement between model-predicted risk and observed risk for classes of subjects. Model evaluation allows researchers to compare their model to other published models for the same population, quantify the model's utility, and check for both lack of fit and overfitting.

Continuous outcomes, modeled by linear regression (see below), are usually evaluated by R^2, the multiple coefficient of determination. It is an overall performance measure reflecting the proportion of variation in response that is explained by the model. Its value ranges from 0 to 1, with larger values being better.

Consider a binary outcome. A model with good discrimination should be able to evaluate the predicted risk of any two subjects such that if one had the outcome and the other did not, higher predictive risk is given to the one who actually had the outcome. The concordance index (C-index or C-statistic) is a popular discrimination tool; others include the integrated discrimination improvement (IDI) and net reclassification index (NRI) (9). Survival outcomes also can use a version of the C-index for discrimination. The C-index can be interpreted as the proportion of discordant subjects who were correctly ranked by the model, in terms of risk. Its value ranges from 0.5, which represents a model that is not better than random guessing, to 1, which represents perfect discrimination.

In addition to appropriate inclusion of covariates, a model's ability to discriminate depends on the inherent "noise" in the outcome. We cannot expect good discrimination of a noisy end point. For example, progression to diabetes is defined by highly variable measures of glucose tolerance (such as fasting glucose level). Even if we knew the exact determinants of glucose intolerance, it would be difficult to discriminate the inaccurate result of a single glucose test. Hence, a good C-index for discrimination of diabetes might be much lower than a good C-index for discrimination of mortality. Discrimination indices are best used for comparison of models of a common end point and common populations.

Calibration is slightly harder to assess. A model with good calibration should produce predicted probabilities that are close to the true risk probabilities. One method of assessment is to compare, via a plot, the mean predicted and mean observed responses in subgroups such as deciles of the predicted probabilities. With this particular subgrouping, the mean observed responses should follow a positive linear trend with the deciles. In such plots, good calibration is determined at the discretion of the investigators, reviewers, and readers. Another tool is the Hosmer–Lemeshow goodness-of-fit test (10), which can identify the lack of fit for a model, such as underfitting or when other assumptions are incorrect.

Both discrimination and calibration must be considered. Below is an illustration, albeit in the extreme, of the pitfalls of describing only a model's discrimination or calibration, but not both. Consider a population where, on average, 30% of patients have the event. If a prognostic model assigns, unrealistically, a predictive probability of 0.8 to all patients without the event and 0.9 to those who actually have the event, the model would have perfect discrimination, or a C-index of 1, because all patients who lacked the outcome had a smaller predicted risk than those having the outcome. However, the average predicted risk is biased high, when it should be 0.3 on average. Thus, it is not well calibrated. Similarly, consider a model for this same outcome where all patients, again unrealistically, have predicted risk of 0.3. Such a model would be perfectly calibrated for the whole population. However, it cannot discriminate among individuals, because they all have equal predictive risk.

A final consideration is that discrimination and calibration measures will be optimistic when calculated on the same dataset from which the model was developed. Therefore, it is common to use a validation dataset or a bootstrap validation process. Performance measures can be calculated in a completely new and independent validation dataset or a small portion of the sample that has been withheld from the initial analysis. For bootstrap validation, the entire modeling process is applied to repeated samples that are drawn from the original dataset, with replacement. Results of the bootstrap samples or validation cohort are more likely to reflect the level of performance that can be expected in future applications of the model to new datasets.

Consider again Roe et al. (2), who identified a predictive model for long-term mortality in older patients with non-ST-segment elevation MI. The researchers chose to randomly divide their sample of 43,239 patients into two cohorts; the first, a derivation cohort of 34,640 (80% of the sample) and the second, a validation cohort of 8,599 (20% of the sample). The predictive model was created using the derivation cohort and evaluated using both the derivation and validation cohorts. They evaluated their model as follows. First, good model discrimination was observed by evaluating the C-indices in the derivation and validation cohorts ($C = 0.754$ and $C = 0.744$, respectively). Second, a calibration plot compared the observed Kaplan–Meier curve for mortality versus predicted probability of mortality at 1 year under their model in the validation cohort. Good calibration of the model was demonstrated, in that the plot of predicted versus observed probabilities was nearly linear with a slope of 1. Finally, the model as a whole was evaluated throughout using the validation cohort. Hazard ratios of the predictive model were nearly identical between the validation cohort and the derivation cohort, and their C-index values were similar.

SPECIFIC MODELS

Linear, logistic, and hazards regression (survival analysis) are common methods used in clinical research to relate covariates and outcomes. Linear regression is the standard method for continuous outcomes. Logistic regression is appropriate for binary outcomes. When binary outcomes are measured prospectively, they are also associated with a time to the event. In this case, either logistic regression or survival analysis can be appropriate. Logistic regression provides a model for outcome/event rates at a specific point in time, for example, the probability of death by 30 days. Hazards regression, typically Cox proportional hazards, addresses time-to-event data and covariate relationships to outcomes over time. In the following, we describe each method in brief using examples from the literature.

Linear Regression

Although an entire course can be devoted to each of the regression techniques in this section, linear regression is the easiest to comprehend. Linear regression relates covariates to the average value of a continuous outcome. It can best be described by an illustrative example.

Once again, consider the analysis by Forman et al. (5). The researchers hypothesized that increased age might relate to worse exercise performance, independent of age-related increases in comorbid conditions. Using cardiopulmonary exercise testing data from HF-ACTION, they assessed the relationship of age to baseline peak oxygen consumption (VO_2) and the ventilation-carbon dioxide production (VE/VCO_2) slope. They created an associative model for each measure of exercise capacity using age and 34 other candidate variables to assess and clarify the relationship of age to exercise capacity.

Peak VO_2 is a continuous outcome (mL/kg/min) measured at a distinct point in time. Thus, a linear regression model was appropriate to identify how age and other covariates are associated with this surrogate for exercise performance. The full results of the study are suppressed here for

TABLE 14–1

Selected independent predictors of peak oxygen consumption (in mL/kg/min) in HF-ACTION: linear regression modeling

Variable	Coefficient	95% Confidence interval	P value
Age			<0.001
≤40 years	0.03	−0.05–0.10	
>40 years	−0.14	−0.16—0.13	
Body mass index[a]	−0.16	−0.18—0.13	<0.001
Female sex (vs. male)	−2.08	−2.43—1.72	<0.001
Race (vs. white)			<0.001
Black	−2.16	−2.53—1.80	
Other	−1.10	−1.81—0.39	

Excerpted from Forman et al. (5).
[a]Increment not reported.

brevity, but they suggest both age and sex as two of the significant predictors of peak VO₂ (Table 14–1).

In a linear regression model, the coefficient for a continuous covariate should be interpreted as the change in the response one would see, on average, for a unit increase in the covariate after adjusting for other covariates in the model. During modeling, age was best fitted with a linear spline. This reflects a nonlinear relationship, in that a single unit change in age did not have a constant relationship to peak VO₂. The linear spline allowed age to have separate linear effects below and above the knot point. In particular, the model suggested that every year of age above 40 would be expected to reduce the predicted peak VO₂ by 0.14 mL/kg/min after adjusting for the other covariates in the model. The researchers were 95% confident that the true decrease for every additional year of age beyond 40 was between −0.16 and −0.13 mL/kg/min; this is the 95% confidence interval (CI). Age ≤ 40 years was not strongly associated with a higher or lower predicted peak VO₂ (0.03; 95% CI, −0.05–0.10) after accounting for other covariates. A test for the overall effect of age suggested that it is a strong predictor of exercise capacity ($P < 0.001$).

The coefficient for a continuous covariate depends greatly on units, and the magnitude can be interpreted only in clinical context. If a researcher wants to know the expected change in response for a 10-unit increase (or any other increase) in a continuous covariate, they can simply multiply the coefficient (and confidence bounds) by 10. Changing the scale in this way has no impact on the P value or significance of association.

For dichotomous covariates, the coefficient is interpreted as the difference in the response one would see, on average, between the two levels of the covariate. For example, after accounting for other covariates in the model, female sex was associated with a predicted peak VO_2 of 2.08 mL/kg/min less compared with male sex, on average. The researchers were 95% confident that the true decrease in exercise capacity among women compared with men was between 1.72 and 2.43 mL/kg/min. The study suggested that sex is also a strong predictor of exercise capacity ($P < 0.001$).

After identifying their initial predictive model, the researchers explored age interactions with comorbid conditions. They sought to see whether the effects of age would be mediated by conditions often correlated with advanced age, noting that "the interaction manifests itself as follows: the relative reductions with age in average peak VO_2 among patients with PAD [peripheral arterial disease] and diabetes were less pronounced than among those without the comorbidities." The researchers used stepwise variable selection to initially identify significant covariates and confounders, and then continued exploring age and comorbidity pathways to exercise capacity. Hence, one might best describe this study as associative, exploring the biological pathways between age, comorbid conditions, and exercise capabilities in the presence of covariates. Among their conclusions: "although VE/VO_2 slope does not change significantly as function of age per se among healthy adults, it becomes relatively steeper in association with diastolic and systolic HF" (5).

Logistic Regression

When a study examines a noncontinuous outcome, a different modeling approach is necessary. Logistic regression is one method for handling binary (yes/no) outcomes. Instead of positing a model for the expected response, researchers use a model for the probability of outcome. Technically, the log-odds (logit) of outcome probability relate linearly to covariates. This particular function has mathematical advantages. The result is that covariate relationships are generally reported in terms of multiplicative changes in the odds of outcome. A statistician will often present a table consisting of odds ratios for each covariate of interest, so that researchers can identify a covariate's effect on the odds of an outcome occurring. We illustrate logistic regression below.

TABLE 14–2

Selected independent predictors of 30-day mortality in patients in the PURSUIT trial

Variable	Odds ratio	95% Confidence interval	P value
Female sex	0.61	0.44–0.84	<0.005
Height			
163 cm (vs. 170 cm)	1.18	1.04–1.33	<0.01
176 cm (vs. 170 cm)	0.87	0.78–0.97	<0.01
Region of enrollment[a]			
Latin America	3.04	1.93–4.78	<0.001
North America	0.90	0.68–1.21	ns
Eastern Europe	1.03	0.74–1.43	ns

Adapted from Boersma et al. (11).
ns, not significant.
[a]Compared with enrollment in Western Europe.

Consider the following example from Boersma and colleagues (11). The researchers were interested in determining what covariates affected the outcomes of death and death or myocardial (re)infarction (MI) within 30 days in the Platelet glycoprotein IIb/IIIa in Unstable angina: Receptor Suppression Using Integrilin Therapy (PURSUIT) study. By appropriately modeling their data, they suggested a subset of factors that should be considered when making clinical decisions.

For the binary outcome of 30-day mortality, logistic regression is well suited to address the study's hypotheses. Select results are available in Table 14–2. In the logistic model, a continuous covariate will have a corresponding odds ratio. The odds ratio is the multiplicative increase in the odds of the outcome one would expect, on average, for a unit increase in the covariate. For a dichotomous covariate, the odds ratio simply provides the odds of the event under one value of the covariate compared with the odds of event under the other value.

The researchers in this study presented specific odds ratios for the median and 25th and 75th percentiles of the distribution of continuous covariates in the study, using the median as a reference. In this study, the odds ratio for height was 0.98, such that for each additional centimeter of height, the odds of mortality decreased by about 2%. Thus, after accounting for other covariates, we would expect an average decrease of 2% in the odds of 30-day death. As shown in Table 14–2, the odds of dying within

30 days for a 163-cm patient are 1.18 times the odds for a 170-cm patient, holding other covariates constant. This is not a separate finding, but a simple calculation from the linear odds ratio, allowing it to be reported for a 7-cm decrease. The researchers were 95% confident that the true increase in the odds ratio was between 1.04 and 1.33 compared with that for the reference group (170 cm).

For dichotomous variables, the interpretation is easier, suggesting that the odds of 30-day death for women were just 0.61 times the odds of 30-day death for men, keeping other covariates constant. There is significant evidence that height and sex ($P < 0.01$ and $P < 0.005$, respectively) are associated with changes in the odds of 30-day death.

As with linear regression, the coefficient for continuous outcomes depends on the scale and magnitude. However, the transition from a 1-unit increment to a 10-unit increment (or any other, such as the 7-unit increment used here) is not as simple as multiplying the odds ratio or CI. Instead, transformations using logarithms and exponentials must be used and should be done with caution. The P value associated with the covariate does not change, however.

The researchers indicated that, "the C-index for the mortality model was 0.814, reflecting good ability to discriminate between patients who did and did not have a fatal outcome" (11). The study did not do a formal analysis of calibration, but during model building, they checked the adequacy of their linearity assumption and applied higher-order splines when necessary, reducing the probability of poor calibration. "A risk-evaluation scheme based on the most important prognostic factors" was developed for 30-day complications [mortality and combined mortality or (re)infarction]. The researchers suggested that "knowledge of the risk profile may affect the clinical decision-making process."

Hazards Regression (Survival Analysis)

When outcomes are associated with time to the event, we are not limited to studying a specific point in time. Instead, we can ask whether the probability of the event tends to be higher over the entire follow-up period. Survival analysis is used to answer this broader question. Just as we used the odds ratio for modeling binary outcomes, there are technical reasons to focus on an alternative quantity that is related to event probabilities, the hazard. A hazard, sometimes called the conditional failure rate, as a function of time is loosely defined as the instantaneous probability of the event occurring at any given time. Event probabilities can be calculated from the hazard, and vice versa.

The most common survival model is the Cox proportional hazards model (12). It relates covariates directly to the hazard of outcome and does not require that we understand the distribution of event times. Technically, this is described as having no assumptions on the baseline hazard. Covariate relationships are generally reported in terms of multiplicative changes in the hazards of outcome, that is, hazard ratios. The hazard ratio tells us whether a change in the covariate shifts the entire hazard curve up or down, corresponding to worse or better survival, respectively.

The Cox proportional hazards regression model assumes that the hazard ratio is constant over time. That is, although the baseline hazard is not modeled and may be changing in some unknown way over time, we assume that covariates have a constant effect on the hazard over time. This is known as the proportional hazards assumption. When statisticians detect a proportional hazards violation, they can employ time-varying coefficients. That is, some covariates may no longer assume proportional hazards over time, but instead the hazard is changed with time. Unfortunately, even detecting a deviation from proportional hazards is not straightforward; further, there is no guarantee of identifying the correct form of a nonproportionality. Thus, caution should be used in interpreting nonproportional hazards except where sufficient clinical knowledge is used to guide the choice of nonproportionality. Further discussion of these topics is beyond the scope of this book, but we refer readers to Fisher and Lin (13) for a thorough explanation.

Despite some concerns, survival analysis and hazards regression remain important and widely used tools to address time-to-event hypotheses. We simply encourage the reader to be mindful of the many potential issues and engage in due diligence. An example below illustrates Cox proportional hazards modeling for interpretation of estimates.

Mahaffey and colleagues provide a good example of hazards regression (14). They sought to establish a predictive model for 1-year survival among patients surviving to 30 days in the Superior Yield of the New strategy of Enoxaparin, Revascularization and GlYcoprotein IIb/IIIa inhibitors (SYNERGY) trial. Using appropriate modeling, they identified important predictors of survival and established a nomogram for 1-year mortality in these patients. Select results of their model are presented in Table 14–3.

The hazard ratio is interpreted as the multiplicative increase in the hazard function per unit increase in a continuous covariate. Similarly, it is the multiplicative increase in the hazard function for one value of a dichotomous variable compared with the other value. Thus, although the baseline hazard is not identified through modeling and might be very complex,

TABLE 14-3

Selected independent predictors of 1-year mortality in patients surviving to 30 days in the SYNERGY trial

Variable	Hazard ratio	95% Confidence interval	P value
Male sex	1.991	1.495–2.652	<0.001
Use of a statin at Day 30	0.607	0.477–0.772	<0.001
Age (per 10-year increase)	1.262	1.078–1.476	0.0037

Adapted from Mahaffey et al. (14).

the hazard ratios indicate whether a change in a covariate shifts the curve up or down in a multiplicative fashion.

The researchers in this study identified several important predictors of survival. Every 10-year increase in age was associated with an average 26.2% increase in the hazard for 1-year mortality, after accounting for other covariates. The 95% CI for this increase was between 7.8% and 47.6% ($P = 0.0037$). Thus, age appears to have a significant effect on 1-year survival among those surviving 30 days. Further, the hazard of 1-year mortality among 30-day survivors was 1.991 (95% CI, 1.495–2.652) times higher for men versus women, holding other covariates constant. That is, increased age and male sex are associated with increased hazard and, equivalently, decreased survival probability.

Again, continuous variables are interpreted in the context of magnitude and scale; here, the authors included age in units of 10 years. As with logistic regression, logarithmic and exponential functions must be used with caution to alter the scale of units employed for the hazard ratio, but the P value does not change.

The authors also presented a nomogram, a chart assigning scores for different levels of predictors so that the sum of the scores predicts the risk of the event. "The scores are associated with probabilities of survival at day 365 (assuming baseline is at day 30) and can thus be used to estimate a subsequent event" (14). The full predictive model had a C-index of 0.822, indicating good predictive discrimination, with a C-index of 0.734 for the reduced model for the nomogram.

Thus far, we have not discussed censored data. Censoring, or a loss of information about outcome, is common in longitudinal follow-up. Censored individuals do not fit into the binary categories of logistic regression.

In such cases, a hazards model might be more appropriate so as to use the available information. Censoring alone is not the indicator of which method to choose, hazards regression can be conducted on data lacking censoring, and logistic regression can be used when mild censoring is present. Rather, both the available data and hypotheses should guide modeling decisions.

Consider again the hazards regression example of Mahaffey and colleagues (14). Although the researchers could have posited a logistic model for the outcome, a hazards model was instead used. This latter model estimates the average effect of each covariate on survival over the interval, as opposed to effects on event rates at a specific point in time. Complete follow-up through 1 year was available for 99.4% of their study patients, indicating that their interests determined the use of a hazards model over a logistic model. The choice was not made because of any substantial censoring.

SUMMARY

Regression requires consideration of both macro and micro problems. For the former, investigators and statisticians should carefully discuss the purpose of the model, deciding whether they are interested in prediction, adjustment, or associative modeling. The model purpose might influence whether variable-selection techniques are used, the degree of model complexity to be considered, and how best to evaluate the model. Careful consideration of these topics can help produce meaningful analyses that adequately address hypotheses to further data-driven medical practice.

REFERENCES

1. Harrell FE. *Regression Modeling Strategies: With Applications to Linear Models, Logistic Regression, and Survival Analysis.* New York, NY: Springer; 2010.
2. Roe MT, et al. Predicting long-term mortality in older patients after non-ST-segment elevation myocardial infarction: the CRUSADE long-term mortality model and risk score. *Am Heart J.* 2011;162(5):875-883.e1.
3. Piccini JP, et al. Antiarrhythmic drug therapy for sustained ventricular arrhythmias complicating acute myocardial infarction. *Crit Care Med.* 2011; 39(1):78-83.

4. Lee KL, et al. Predictors of 30-day mortality in the era of reperfusion for acute myocardial infarction. Results from an international trial of 41,021 patients. GUSTO-I Investigators. *Circulation.* 1995;91(6):1659-1668.
5. Forman DE, et al. Relationship of age and exercise performance in patients with heart failure: the HF-ACTION study. *Am Heart J.* 2009;158 (suppl): S6-S15.
6. Tibshirani R. Regression shrinkage and selection via the LASSO. *J R Stat Soc Series B.* 1996;58:267-288.
7. Boos DD, Stefanski LA, Wu Y. Fast FSR variable selection with applications to clinical trials. *Biometrics.* 2009;65(3):692-700.
8. Tibshirani R. The lasso method for variable selection in the Cox model. *Stat Med.* 1997;16(4):385-395.
9. Pencina MJ, D'Agostino RB Sr, D'Agostino RB Jr, Vasan RS. Evaluating the added predictive ability of a new marker: from area under the ROC curve to reclassification and beyond. *Stat Med.* 2008;27(2):157-172; discussion 207-212.
10. Hosmer DW, Lemeshow S. *Applied Logistic Regression.* New York, NY: Wiley; 2000.
11. Boersma E, et al. Predictors of outcome in patients with acute coronary syndromes without persistent ST-segment elevation. Results from an international trial of 9461 patients. The PURSUIT Investigators. *Circulation.* 2000; 101(22):2557-2567.
12. Cox DR. Regression models and life tables (with discussion). *J R Stat Soc Series B.* 1972;34:187-220.
13. Fisher LD, Lin DY. Time-dependent covariates in the Cox proportional-hazards regression model. *Annu Rev Public Health.* 1999;20:145-157.
14. Mahaffey KW, et al. Prediction of one-year survival in high-risk patients with acute coronary syndromes: results from the SYNERGY trial. *J Gen Intern Med.* 2008;23(3):310-316.

CHAPTER FIFTEEN

Analytical Methods of Addressing Confounding

Eric M. Reyes and Laine E. Thomas

INTRODUCTION

Chapter 13 discussed many of the obstacles inherent in the analysis of data from observational studies, with bias due to confounding arguably the largest of these concerns. Confounding can be seen as an issue of "mistaken identity," in which the cause of an observed effect is attributed to the wrong party. As an example, consider a cohort study undertaken to assess the efficacy of a treatment. In this cohort, younger people are more likely to receive the treatment and are less likely to experience the outcome of interest (Figure 15–1). If a treatment effect is observed, it is unclear whether the observed effect is due to the treatment or to the younger age of the patients receiving the treatment. That is, age and treatment are said to be confounded; equivalently, age is said to be a confounder. Formally, a confounder is any variable related to *both* the outcome of interest and the treatment under study. In our example, age affects *both* the event rate *and* which treatment the person receives.

Throughout this chapter, we will refer to nonrandomized "treatment." This term is not restricted to a medication; it can refer to a medical procedure or any variable of interest. The key characteristic of this "treatment" is that it was *not* assigned at random during the study. To facilitate discussion, we will typically consider a binary treatment; that is, patients can be divided into two treatment (or exposure) groups. Everything presented in this chapter can be generalized to the case of multiple treatment groups.

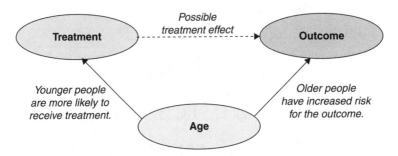

FIGURE 15–1. Illustration of confounding. In this hypothetical scenario, age is a confounder because it is related to both the treatment of interest and the outcome under study.

Whenever the exposure to a "treatment" is not due to randomization (such as in an observational study), confounding is likely. If we fail to address the confounding when conducting the analysis, we could mistakenly attribute an observed difference to the treatment under study when, in actuality, the difference is due to a second factor. In this chapter, we introduce several analytical approaches commonly used to address confounding. We also discuss the clinical assumptions underlying each method and common pitfalls to avoid.

REGRESSION ADJUSTMENT

Suppose a patient with a recent diagnosis of hypertension asks for a treatment recommendation. Should the physician make this recommendation without meeting with the patient? Or would he or she first want to consider the patient's history, collect vital signs, etc.? This latter approach— making treatment decisions *given* certain patient characteristics—suggests a "conditional" approach to addressing confounding. That is, if treatment decisions are made conditionally, perhaps the treatment effect we are interested in estimating is the effect given other patient characteristics. This is the motivation behind regression adjustment. Although the details of regression models were covered in *Chapter 14*, we will briefly consider how a regression model can be used to adjust for confounding.

The concept is straightforward: include the treatment and any potential confounders (variables related to both treatment and outcome) in a regression model. The estimated treatment effect in this multivariable regression model is then adjusted for the confounders included in the

TABLE 15-1

Unadjusted results from a study investigating the benefit of emergency medical system (EMS) transport in patients with acute myocardial infarction

	Self-transport ($n = 15049$)	EMS transport ($n = 22585$)	P value
Minutes from symptom onset to hospital arrival	120 (60–285)	89 (57–163)	<0.001

Values are summarized as medians (25th–75th percentiles).
Adapted from Mathews et al. (1).

model. Identifying all potential confounders is not straightforward, however. Because the issue of identifying confounders underlies each of the methods presented, we will return to it at the end of this chapter. For now, let us assume we know which variables contribute to the confounding.

Mathews et al. (1) investigated the benefit of using emergency medical services (EMS) transport versus self-transport in patients who were having acute myocardial infarction (MI). The authors first compared the "raw" or unadjusted times from symptom onset to hospital arrival between patients transported by EMS and those transporting themselves (Table 15–1), finding that people transported by EMS arrived at the hospital significantly earlier after their symptoms began than did patients who transported themselves. They then repeated the comparison after adjusting for sociodemographic factors (including age and ethnicity) and clinical factors (including systolic blood pressure and prior stroke) that each were associated with the use of EMS transport. After multivariable adjustment, EMS-transported patients were still about twice as likely as self-transported patients to arrive at the hospital within 120 minutes after symptom onset ($P < 0.001$). The logistic model for the probability of arriving at the hospital within 120 minutes after symptom onset included both the mode of transportation used by the patient and all confounding variables. The odds ratio associated with the mode of transportation from this multivariable model is the value reported by the authors.

The results suggest that *among two patients with common values for all confounding variables*, those who use EMS transport arrive at the hospital earlier, on average, than those who transport themselves. Notice that this result is interpreted as conditional on the knowledge of other variables.

One pitfall common in regression analysis is extrapolation—assuming the treatment effect is valid for a patient who is not represented in the sample. Once numerous variables are entered into a model, it can be difficult to determine when extrapolation is occurring. For example, in the EMS study above, the result might not apply to a 75-year-old white man who has not had a prior stroke if no such individual was included in the sample. Additionally, the relationship between confounders and outcome must be modeled correctly, including nonlinearity and even interactions. Although a simple model can suffice, there is no guarantee that it does, and conclusions could be erroneous if the model is not accurate.

STRATIFICATION

Intuitively, if we restrict our analysis to a subgroup of patients who are similar with respect to the confounding variables, then any remaining treatment effect should not be biased. Thus, we might consider doing a separate analysis in each of these subgroups. Such a subgroup analysis, however, prevents us from using all available data. Stratification reconciles these two objectives by combining the information from each subgroup to develop a better estimate of the treatment effect. This approach has three steps: (1) divide the sample into groups (or "strata") that have similar values of the confounders, (2) run the analysis in each group, and (3) combine the results to obtain an overall estimate of the treatment effect. This approach is valid if the treatment effect is believed to be similar within each group, and there are no remaining differences between patients that could confound treatment within the strata.

Consider a hypothetical study in which investigators use an existing trial database to compare the efficacy of two treatments in reducing the rate of MI 30 days after percutaneous coronary intervention (PCI). The data include patients for whom treatment was assigned at the discretion of the physician. It is known that diabetic patients were more likely to receive Treatment A, but there were no other characteristics associated with treatment. We believe that the treatment should have the same effect in diabetic patients as in nondiabetic patients. To adjust for the confounding via stratification, we compute the treatment effect for diabetic and nondiabetic patients separately; then we combine the results to get an overall treatment effect. This process is illustrated in Figure 15–2.

Note that this is *not* a subgroup analysis. The effect within each stratum is not reported separately; the stratification is used only to adjust for

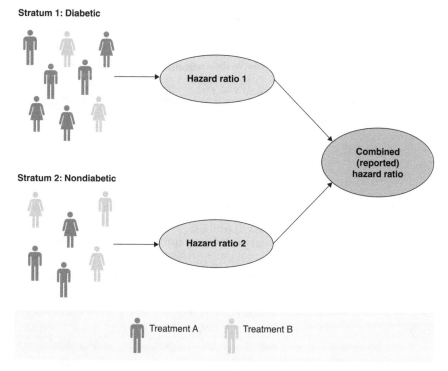

FIGURE 15–2. Illustration of stratification. The sample is divided into groups of patients who share similar values of the confounding variables. Estimates of the treatment effect within each group are combined to form an overall treatment effect.

the confounding, and the final pooled estimate is of singular interest. Although stratification is intuitive, it can become complicated to implement as the number of confounders grows, because we need to identify multiple patients assigned to each treatment that will fall within a given strata. In the example above, we identified diabetic patients who were assigned Treatment A and diabetic patients who were assigned Treatment B (similarly for nondiabetics). However, suppose we stratified on diabetic status, sex, race, and age. It can be very difficult to find multiple patients taking Treatment A and multiple patients taking Treatment B who are diabetic, female, Caucasian, and more than 65 years old.

As with regression analysis, the estimate obtained from stratification is conditionally interpreted as the effect among individuals with common values for all strata variables. The conditional approach is powerful, but the results do not mimic those of a clinical trial. Clinical trials assess the "marginal" effect— the treatment effect that we might expect to see on average in the population.

It is natural to then question which interpretation is best, conditional or marginal. When the goal of a study is to establish that a treatment effect exists, a distinction between these interpretations is rarely made. Although the resulting estimate may differ depending on the method chosen, the direction of the effect and its significance are not likely to change. Therefore, the effect of a treatment can be established using either approach. However, care should be given to the desired interpretation before a method is chosen.

MATCHING

We can think of extending stratification in such a way that exactly two patients (one from each treatment group) fall into each stratum. This leads to matching. As the name implies, matching involves pairing patients in one treatment group with those in the other who are similar. Patients should be matched with respect to confounding variables. That is, each patient in one treatment group is paired with a patient in the other treatment group who has similar values for the confounding variables. Matching can be a part of the data collection, or it can take place afterward; however, it is much easier to ensure good results in the former case. Thus, it is important to have a statistician involved during the early phases of the study design and data collection.

Suppose you would like to use data collected in a registry to compare the efficacy of two treatments in reducing mortality at 30 days after treatment. You have identified patients who received Treatment A, the treatment of interest. Further, you know that sex and diabetes status are potential confounders and would like to account for these via matching. For each of the patients who received Treatment A, you must identify a patient from the registry who received Treatment B (the competitor) who is of the same sex and diabetes status. This process will create two groups that are similar *with respect to the variables used in the matching process* (sex and diabetes in this case), as illustrated in Figure 15–3. Differences between the matched groups cannot be attributable to sex or diabetes, because the groups are similar in these features. When no other confounders exist, differences must be attributable to treatment.

Similar to stratification, matching can become difficult to implement as the number of confounders increases. For example, whereas it is easy to identify two subjects with similar values of sex and diabetes status, it can be impossible to identify two subjects with similar values of sex, diabetes status, age, race, ejection fraction, creatinine clearance, and systolic blood pressure. Matching also can result in the exclusion of many patients; those

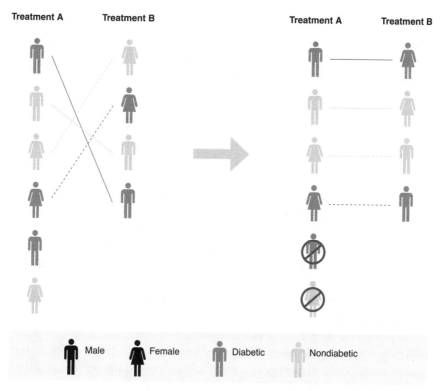

FIGURE 15–3. Illustration of matching. Similar patients, with respect to defined characteristics, are paired before analyzing the data. This makes the treatment groups similar. In this example, the confounding variables used in the matching process were sex and diabetes status at baseline. Patients who are not matched are excluded from the study.

who do not have a counterpart in the other treatment group are excluded from analysis (see Figure 15–3).

If matching is chosen, it must be accounted for in any analysis performed. There are different ways to account for matching, but the key is to remember that matched pairs are no longer independent and should be analyzed like correlated data. Methods such as generalized estimating equations can be used and maintain the marginal interpretation.

PROPENSITY SCORES

Currently, the most popular methods for addressing confounding involve propensity scores (2–4). In an observational study, many factors determine which treatment a patient receives. We have already seen that older patients might receive the treatment of interest more often than younger patients, or diabetic patients might tend to receive the treatment of interest more often. The idea behind a propensity score is to summarize all the information about a subject's confounding variables into a single value—the likelihood of receiving the treatment of interest. For example, a subject with a propensity score of 0.5 would be equally likely to have received either treatment, whereas a subject with a propensity score of 0.9 is almost certain to have received the treatment of interest, based on his or her characteristics.

Methods that involve propensity scores require two analyses: (1) constructing a model to estimate the propensity score for each individual and (2) using the propensity score to adjust for confounding when estimating the treatment effect. (When developing a model for the propensity to receive the treatment of interest, a simple model may suffice, but there is no guarantee that it does, and conclusions could be erroneous if the model is not accurate.)

What variables should be used to estimate the propensity score? All confounding variables (anything related to both the outcome and the treatment) should be placed in the propensity score model. At this point, however, the outcome itself should *not* be used. If we think about it, this makes sense; only variables that were known before the patient received the treatment would have influenced which treatment the patient received. Because the outcome occurred after the patient was assigned the treatment, it should have had no bearing on which treatment the patient was likely to receive.

Once the model has been fitted, we use it to estimate a propensity score for each individual. Once we have a propensity score for each individual, we can use it to adjust for confounding in one of several ways.

Stratification

Instead of stratifying subjects based on a set of confounders as previously discussed, we can stratify subjects based on the propensity score. Subjects can be placed into five groups that have similar propensity scores; for example, one group could be the 20% of subjects with the largest propensity scores. The analysis is then conducted within each stratum, and the results combined, to obtain an overall estimate of the treatment effect (Figure 15–4). Despite stratifying on the propensity score alone, covariates become approximately balanced across the treatment groups within strata and can therefore no longer be confounders. This approach is motivated by

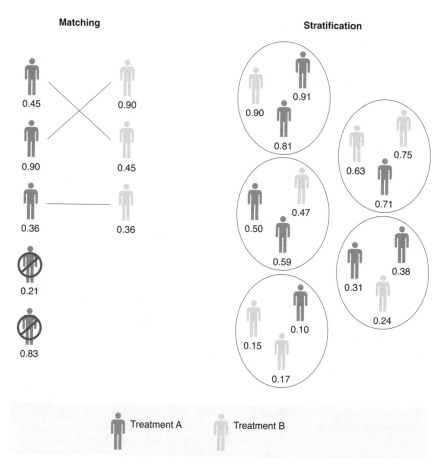

FIGURE 15–4. Illustration of matching and stratification via propensity scores. The sequences proceed just as before, except that grouping is based on the value of each subject's propensity score.

the following intuition: if we collected all subjects with a similar propensity score (similar probability of receiving treatment) in the world, then among these patients each is equally likely to receive one treatment or another. Thus, we would expect the covariates to be equally balanced within this group (similar to a clinical trial).

Matching

Similar to stratifying on the propensity score, we could match subjects based on their propensity score. Pairing patients with similar values of the propensity score will create two treatment groups that are balanced with respect to the variables included in the propensity model. Again, it often happens that no match for a particular patient is found; this can result in the exclusion of many patients from the study (Figure 15–4).

Weintraub et al. (5) used data from a large registry to compare the long-term mortality of patients undergoing PCI with those undergoing coronary artery bypass grafting (CABG). Because patients were not randomized to the chosen procedure, confounding was a concern. The authors adjusted for this confounding using propensity scores via inverse probability weighting (IPW) (discussed in the next section); as a sensitivity analysis, they reanalyzed the data-matching subjects based on the propensity score. First, they constructed a logistic model to estimate the propensity for a subject to undergo CABG based on several patient and hospital characteristics. The accuracy of this propensity model is critical if the results are to be trusted; as a result, the authors developed a very flexible model. Subjects who underwent PCI were then matched to subjects with a similar propensity score who underwent CABG. Of the 103549 patients undergoing PCI and the 86244 patients undergoing CABG, only 43084 patients in each group were matched to a subject in the opposing group. That is, less than half of the subjects in the study were retained for this sensitivity analysis. This is a large drawback of matching. The results of the sensitivity analysis confirmed their primary findings: by 4 years after surgery, the probability of survival was significantly higher for patients undergoing CABG.

Inverse Probability Weighting

Inverse weighting via propensity scores is commonly used in outcomes research. It is an alternative to matching and stratification when using the propensity score to adjust for confounding. The idea is to allow each person to represent both him or herself and those who are very similar *but received the other treatment* (again, with respect to the confounding variables taken into account through the propensity score). That is, if Bob received Treatment A, we want to use Bob to represent other patients who are similar to him but who received Treatment B. In IPW, each person represents $(1/X)$ people, where X is the probability of receiving the treatment actually received. If the patient received the treatment of interest, X is their propensity score; if the patient received the other treatment, X is 1 minus the propensity score. For example, suppose Bob received Treatment A (the treatment of interest) and has a propensity score of 0.25 and Karen

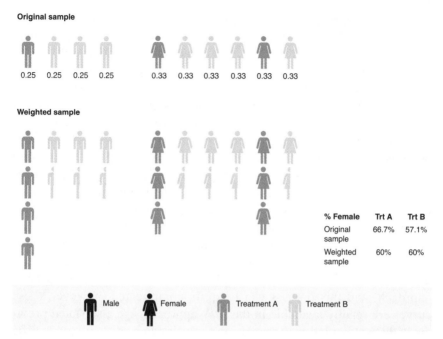

FIGURE 15-5. Illustration of inverse probability weighting **(IPW)** via propensity scores. Here, sex is the only confounder, with men having a 0.25 probability of receiving Treatment **(Trt)** A, and women, a 0.33 probability of receiving Treatment A. After inverse weighting, the sample is balanced with respect to sex.

received Treatment B (the other treatment) and has a propensity score of 0.33, Bob will represent himself and three other people (1/0.25 = 4) and Karen will represent herself and half of another person (1/(1−0.33) = 1.5). Weighting in this fashion makes our sample resemble what we would expect to see in a clinical trial (Figure 15−5). Confounding is therefore addressed by running the analysis we would have conducted in a clinical trial on the weighted sample.

As previously discussed, Weintraub et al. (5) reported the results of an observational study comparing the long-term mortality of patients undergoing PCI and CABG. The authors identified 29 patient-level and hospital-level confounders for which to adjust, including age, sex, race, body mass index, glomerular filtration rate, renal failure, average hospital volume of PCI, and hospital location (rural or urban). Using the weighted sample, the authors presented Kaplan–Meier survival curves showing that by 4 years, patients undergoing CABG had significantly higher survival compared with those undergoing PCI.

When designing the analysis, the authors chose to adjust for confounding via IPW as opposed to regression modeling. It is worth asking why IPW might be preferred to a regression-adjusted approach. Glynn et al. provide substantial discussion of this topic (6). Neither method is inherently superior; however, there were some practical advantages to choosing IPW in this situation. As we have stated, for both the regression-adjusted and IPW approach, a model must be accurately specified; an incorrect model can lead to erroneous conclusions. With a large number of confounders (29 in this case), it might be very difficult to correctly specify either the outcome model (regression adjustment) or the propensity model (IPW approach); however, you might have more confidence in your ability to specify a model for determining which treatment a person receives than in your ability to specify the model for the outcome, given that the former is dictated by clinician expertise. The authors presented adjusted survival curves as part of the results. There are several definitions for constructing these adjusted curves under the regression approach, and this process can be quite complicated; however, these curves are readily available in the IPW approach. We also stated previously that extrapolation in regression analysis can be difficult to identify. Although extrapolation is a concern with propensity score models, it is often much easier to see. Both the IPW and regression-adjusted approach yield valid results; interpretation and feasibility often dictate which method is preferred.

CHOOSING CONFOUNDERS

Thus far, we have assumed that we know what variables are confounders. We now address how this list is chosen in practice. Ideally, the list of variables should be driven by physician expertise. We should look at the treatment under study and ask, "what characteristics do physicians (or patients) use to determine which treatment a patient will receive, and which of these is believed to affect the outcome?" Any variables identified by this question should be considered confounders. This means that a new list must be created for *each* treatment–outcome combination analyzed. We should not use the same confounders identified for studying the effect of statin use on mortality as when studying the effect of statin use on progression to diabetes, for example. When the outcome of interest (or the treatment under study) changes, the list of confounders should be reevaluated.

When no clinical expertise is available, we often settle on a conservative approach. Recall that confounders are associated with both treatment and outcome. Failing to include all confounders can lead to biased estimates (the mistaken identity issue); on the other hand, falsely claiming that a variable is a confounder will make estimates inefficient (wide confidence intervals). Because bias is often the greater concern, a conservative approach would include all variables associated with the outcome (if possible), which is often an easier list to generate.

There is no way to ensure that all confounders have been identified. This must be assumed when performing the analysis. Some diagnostic tools are useful in guiding this process, however. After accounting for the confounders, the two treatment groups should look similar (with respect to the chosen confounders); that is, after weighting (for example) the two treatment groups should appear as if they were from a randomized trial. A lack of balance between the two groups can indicate that a confounder has been omitted; however, caution should be exercised because balance between the groups does *not* indicate that all confounders have been identified.

BLACK BOX

These analytical procedures, especially those involving propensity scores, can seem like a black box. There is a temptation to claim that the results are "adjusted" and therefore reliable. However, as with any other procedure, these methods require certain assumptions to be met. We now discuss a few of the assumptions that underlie each of the methods discussed above.

Observed Confounders

No method is magic. We cannot adjust for variables we do not observe (capture). Therefore, when designing an observational study, think carefully about the potential confounders and be sure they are collected during the study. Be sure to list in the methods section of any study report the list of confounders used to create adjusted analyses, and list in the limitations section any potential confounders that were not collected. Again, we stress that if the propensity score model is not correctly specified (for example, a confounder is omitted), the results may not be reliable.

Independent Responses

The stable unit treatment value assumption (SUTVA) says that a subject's outcome depends only on that patient's characteristics and treatment received; it does not depend on the outcome of other subjects. This is generally true in cardiovascular clinical trials, but it should be kept in mind. Consider a trial investigating an infectious disease; in this instance, a patient's risk of contracting the disease relates to how many other people have the disease—especially if family members are all participants in the study.

No Complete Confounding

Suppose the inclusion criteria for a trial required that all women of childbearing age use birth control to prevent pregnancy. Data from this trial could never be used to address whether women using birth control are at higher risk for the primary outcome because we have no control group; all women were using contraceptives. This may seem obvious, but once many confounders are being considered, it can become subtle. For example, were there elderly diabetic men with a history of MI in both treatment arms? If there is no chance that a patient with a given set of characteristics could have received a specific treatment, complete confounding is present. There is no way to handle such cases without making strong assumptions.

Marginal Interpretation

When done correctly, marginal approaches are designed to estimate the causal effect of "treatment" when covariates are balanced (as with randomization). This concept depends on our ability to assign treatment over and above existing characteristics (e.g., smoking status, medical procedures, and drugs). When the variable of interest is not actually an assignable action but some inherent characteristic, the value of a marginal approach is less clear. What would be the causal effect of male versus female sex, if these groups could be balanced on all other characteristics (weight, height, hormone levels)? Such a world does not exist. Some characteristics are inextricably linked to sex, so it is unclear why we would frame the question this way. For this reason, methods such as propensity scores are questionable when the goal is to study a fixed attribute. Instead, we often use regression to account for various characteristics and evaluate whether any additional association remains with a particular variable of interest (i.e., sex) after accounting for weight, height, and hormone levels.

Similarly, propensity scores adjust for confounding by creating balance. Ultimately, we expect the results to be quite similar, though the propensity approach is philosophically questionable.

INSTRUMENTAL VARIABLES

Before closing this chapter, we briefly discuss the instrumental variables (IV) framework (7). For each of the methods previously described, identification of confounders is paramount; further, each method requires the assumption that confounders were measured. The IV framework attempts to estimate the unconfounded effect of treatment on outcome, bypassing confounders. Randomization is an ideal example. In a randomized clinical trial, the treatment being assigned can be thought of as the result of a coin flip (Figure 15–6). Although variables other than the treatment might

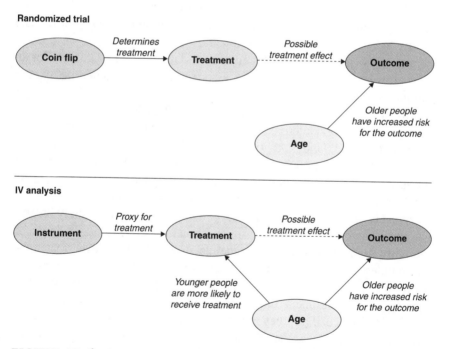

FIGURE 15–6. Comparison of instrumental variables (IV) and randomized trial frameworks. In an IV analysis, the instrument must be associated with the outcome ONLY through the treatment. Notice that although age is confounded with treatment, the instrument is not associated with anything that is related to outcome (other than treatment).

affect the outcome, we get a clear look at the treatment effect because the distribution of confounding variables is balanced across randomized groups.

More generally, an instrument is a variable associated with receiving treatment, but not otherwise associated with outcome and hence not associated with confounders. Suppose we identify a patient characteristic that predicts treatment assignment in an observational study. If this characteristic does not relate to the outcome (except through its effect on determining treatment) and does not relate to other variables affecting outcome, then this characteristic is called an instrument. Notice that in Figure 15–6, we can think of drawing a straight line directly from the instrument to the outcome going *through* the treatment, and that age, although a confounder for treatment, is not related to the instrument. Thus, if the analysis was based on the instrument instead of the treatment, we could bypass the confounder (age, in this case) and the effect would be a proxy for the effect of treatment.

This may sound very similar to the propensity-score method, in that we are trying to find something that predicts treatment. The key difference is in what is used for the prediction. For propensity scores, we use the confounders—the variables related to both outcome and treatment. For an IV analysis, the instrument is *not* associated with the outcome, except through treatment.

In an IV analysis, we are estimating the effect for the compliers—the ideal patients who would receive treatment only if the instrument favors it, but not otherwise. Under additional assumptions, this effect is then generalized to the entire population as a marginal effect. Similar to the other marginal methods described above, an IV analysis is trying to estimate what we would have seen in a clinical trial.

Xian et al. (8) reported the results of a large observational study investigating the association between hospitalization in a stroke center and reduced mortality in patients with acute ischemic stroke. They believed that some confounders were not measured, preventing the use of the techniques described above. However, they were able to identify a characteristic they thought was an instrument: differential distance. Differential distance "is the additional distance, if any, beyond the nearest hospital to reach a stroke center." The hypothesis was that if patients were closer to a nondesignated hospital, EMS personnel might not have risked the additional time needed to transport them to a stroke center. Note that this instrument should have no relationship to age, sex, or other characteristics associated with mortality (the primary outcome). The only characteristic this instrument should affect is treatment assignment (stroke center or nondesignated hospital). However, such a statement is an assumption and cannot be verified rigorously. Also note that this characteristic *preceded* treatment assignment, preventing the treatment from having caused the observed instrument. After using the instrument as a proxy for random treatment assignment, the study found that "admission to a designated stroke center was associated with a 2.5% absolute reduction in 30-day all-cause mortality" ($P < 0.001$).

Another excellent example of IV methods is provided by Stukel and colleagues (9), who compare the methods described above as applied to the comparison of medical versus invasive treatment for acute MI. D'Agostino et al. refer to this example and provide insightful commentary (10).

SUMMARY

If the treatment of interest was not randomly assigned, confounding exists and must be addressed to prevent obtaining biased estimates. The chosen approach should be governed by the type of estimate desired: conditional (given other characteristics) or marginal (clinical trial interpretation). In considering approaches, consider the number of confounders. Regardless of the method selected, remember—one can adjust only for what was collected. Properly adjusting for confounding can result in very meaningful research that can pave the way for future clinical trials.

REFERENCES

1. Mathews R, et al. Use of emergency medical service transport among patients with ST-segment-elevation myocardial infarction: findings from the National Cardiovascular Data Registry Acute Coronary Treatment Intervention Outcomes Network Registry-Get With The Guidelines. *Circulation*. 2011;124(2): 154-163.
2. Austin PC. A critical appraisal of propensity-score matching in the medical literature between 1996 and 2003. *Stat Med*. 2008;27(12):2037-2049.
3. Cavuto S, Bravi F, Grassi MC, Apolone G. Propensity score for the analysis of observational data: an introduction and an illustrative example. *Drug Dev Res*. 2006;67(3):208-216.
4. Rubin DB. Estimating causal effects from large data sets using propensity scores. *Ann Intern Med*. 1997;127(8 Pt 2):757-763.
5. Weintraub WS, et al. Comparative effectiveness of revascularization strategies. *N Engl J Med*. 2012;366(16):1467-1476.

6. Glynn RJ, Schneeweiss S, Stürmer T. Indications for propensity scores and review of their use in pharmacoepidemiology. *Basic Clin Pharmacol Toxicol*. 2006;98(3):253-259.

7. Rassen JA, Brookhart MA, Glynn RJ, Mittleman MA, Schneeweiss S. Instrumental variables I: instrumental variables exploit natural variation in nonexperimental data to estimate causal relationships. *J Clin Epidemiol*. 2009; 62(12):1226-1232.

8. Xian Y, et al. Association between stroke center hospitalization for acute ischemic stroke and mortality. *JAMA*. 2011;305(4):373-380.

9. Stukel TA, et al. Analysis of observational studies in the presence of treatment selection bias: effects of invasive cardiac management on AMI survival using propensity score and instrumental variable methods. *JAMA*. 2007;297(3): 278-285.

10. D'Agostino RB Jr, D'Agostino RB Sr. Estimating treatment effects using observational data. *JAMA*. 2007;297(3):314-316.

CHAPTER SIXTEEN

Lessons from Notable Examples in Observational Research

Zubin J. Eapen

INTRODUCTION

The imperative for sound clinical research continues to increase in response to the demand for evidence-based, guideline-driven medicine. To increase the quality of health care and improve clinical decision-making, innumerable studies have contributed to a hierarchy of evidence for each disease state. The randomized trial often stands at the pinnacle of this hierarchy, yielding the highest level of evidence through a blinded experiment of an intervention or treatment. Preceding observational studies often generate the equipoise and hypotheses for randomized trials. In other instances, observational research can be the best vehicle for generating the evidence. The experimentation inherent in a randomized trial might be unnecessary, inappropriate, or even impossible under certain circumstances. Political, legal, and ethical barriers also can prohibit randomized trials. Increasingly, the costs of large trials are creating another barrier to generating randomized evidence, reducing incentives for funding the head-to-head trials needed to understand the real-world effectiveness of novel therapies. It is therefore important, in the context of the emerging field of comparative effectiveness research, to understand the value and appropriateness of observational research versus

	Trials	Registries/ Observational studies
Strengths	Define treatment effects Define safety Higher data quality	"Real-life" applications Population outcomes
Weaknesses	Few data regarding long-term effects Lack generalizability Expensive Safety in high-risk populations	Unreliable inferences about treatment effects Lower data quality

FIGURE 16–1. Strengths and weaknesses of clinical trials versus observational studies.

randomized trials in answering different clinical questions (Figure 16–1). Prior observational studies, both successes and failures, can inform future efforts in comparative effectiveness.

VALUE OF OBSERVATIONAL RESEARCH IN THE HIERARCHY OF EVIDENCE

Hierarchies of evidence are not the same across disease states. In prevalent conditions with substantial morbidity and mortality, public and private resources are often devoted to generating high-quality evidence from randomized trials. However, even in cardiovascular disease, the leading cause of death in the United States, guideline recommendations are largely developed from lower-level sources of evidence or expert opinion (1,2).

In unstudied subgroups, observational data often serve as guidance for clinical decision-making. For example, age is a significant determinant of outcomes for patients with acute coronary syndromes (ACS), and almost 25% of percutaneous coronary interventions (PCIs) in contemporary practice are performed in patients older than 75 years (3,4). However, most clinical trials exclude such patients. From 1991 to 2000, patients older than 75 years accounted for only 9% of trial enrollment, despite accounting for 37% of all patients with myocardial infarction (MI) in the United States (5). In place of randomized clinical trials, large clinical registries have provided much of the information that informs treatment patterns for this growing subgroup of patients undergoing coronary revascularization.

The American Heart Association (AHA) 2007 scientific statement on acute coronary care in the elderly (6) relied on the National Registry of Myocardial Infarction (NRMI), the Global Registry of Acute Coronary Events (GRACE) (7), and the Can Rapid risk stratification of Unstable angina patients Suppress ADverse outcomes with Early implementation of the ACC/AHA guidelines? (CRUSADE) national quality improvement initiative (8) to determine in-hospital and long-term outcomes for elderly patients (Table 16–1) (6). Complementing data from randomized trials (9–13), these registries indicated that elderly patients with ACS are at high risk for death and other adverse events and therefore derive greater benefit from revascularization than do younger patients. Observational data from these registries will continue to complement trial data by monitoring the safety and efficacy of ACS therapies in the elderly to better understand their utility in this understudied subgroup.

DISCREPANCIES BETWEEN OBSERVATIONAL RESEARCH AND RANDOMIZED TRIALS

The results of clinical trials often diverge from observational data. For example, prior observational studies established total plasma homocysteine level as an independent cardiovascular risk factor (14–18). These findings were disproven by subsequent randomized studies, however, which showed that lowering homocysteine levels had no effect on recurrent cardiovascular disease in patients with acute MI or on major cardiovascular events in patients with vascular disease (19,20). Similarly, observational data suggested that vitamin E supplementation was associated with a reduced risk of coronary artery disease (CAD) and progression of coronary artery lesions (21–23). Subsequent randomized data indicated that long-term vitamin E supplementation did not affect cardiovascular outcomes (24).

The discrepancy between observational research and randomized trials is well illustrated by the case of hormone replacement therapy

TABLE 16–1

Data sources for the American Heart Association's scientific statement on acute coronary care in elderly patients

Source	Enrollment years	n	Age ≥75 years (%)	Regions	Randomized treatment(s)
VIGOUR (pooled)					
GUSTO-IIb (9)	1994–1996	8011	19.5	9 countries	Hirudin vs. heparin
PARAGON-A (10)	1995–1995	2282	19.1	20 countries	GPI (lamifiban) vs. heparin
PARAGON-B (11)	1997–1999	5225	17.8	26 countries	GPI (lamifiban) vs. placebo
PURSUIT (12)	1995–1997	10,948	14.6	28 countries	GPI (eptifibatide) vs. placebo
GUSTO IV-ACS (13)	1998–2000	7800	22.7	24 countries	GPI (abciximab) vs. placebo
NRMI 2–4 (6)	1994–2003	10,76,796	38.3	United States	NSTE MI registry
GRACE (7)	1999–2004	11,968	31.6	14 countries	NSTE ACS registry
CRUSADE (8)	2001–2003	56,963	39.9	United States	NSTE ACS QI initiative

ACS, acute coronary syndromes; GPI, glycoprotein IIb/IIIa inhibitor; MI, myocardial infarction; NSTE, non-ST-segment elevation; QI, quality improvement.
Adapted from Alexander et al. (6), with permission.

(HRT). After first receiving approval for the treatment of menopausal symptoms, HRT subsequently was found in numerous observational studies to have potentially beneficial effects in a variety of conditions. A 1992 meta-analysis in the *Annals of Internal Medicine* (25) recapitulated many of the observed benefits in observational studies, concluding that HRT should probably be recommended for women who have had a hysterectomy, who have CAD, or who are at high risk for CAD. Several meta-analyses, including the 1992 report, drew from the Nurses' Health Study, in which 12,1700 female nurses aged 30–55 years completed mailed questionnaires about postmenopausal hormone use and medical history (26). The study estimated the relative risk (RR) of CAD with the use of HRT at 0.61 overall (95% confidence interval [CI], 0.52–0.71), with an RR of 0.55 (95% CI, 0.45–0.68) for women taking estrogen alone and 0.64 (95% CI, 0.49–0.85) for women taking estrogen plus progestin.

This benefit of HRT in women with or at risk for CAD was not ultimately seen in the Women's Health Initiative (WHI), a randomized trial conducted from 1992 to 2007 (27). A complex trial of multiple strategies for prevention of common causes of morbidity and mortality in women, it was designed to test the efficacy of a low-fat diet, HRT, and calcium and vitamin D supplementation. The study's hypothesis was that HRT would reduce the risk of CAD and bone fractures (although potentially increasing the risk of breast cancer). Over 15 years, WHI randomized 16,608 postmenopausal women aged 50–76 years who had not undergone hysterectomy to receive either combined estrogen and progestin or placebo. In a second study, it randomized 10,739 postmenopausal women aged 50–79 years who *had* undergone hysterectomy to receive estrogen alone or placebo.

The first study was terminated prematurely due to a statistically significantly increased risk of breast cancer with combination HRT. The second study was also terminated prematurely because the trial showed neither cardioprotective benefits nor increased breast cancer risk, with an unacceptably high risk of stroke. Compared with previously observed benefits for CAD in nonrandomized studies, WHI showed a statistically significant increase in the unadjusted rate of CAD among women treated with estrogen plus progestin (RR versus placebo, 1.29; 95% CI, 1.02–1.63) (Table 16–2) (25–32). The WHI finding of an increased risk for breast cancer, on the other hand, was concordant with both preceding epidemiological studies and data from nonhuman primates (33).

TABLE 16-2

Results from observational studies of combined estrogen–progestin replacement therapy and the Women's Health Initiative

Disease	Relative risk (95% confidence interval)	
	Observational studies[a]	Women's Health Initiative[b]
Breast cancer		1.26 (1.00–1.59)
<5 years	1.15	–
≥5 years	1.53	–
Colorectal cancer	0.66 (0.59–0.74)	0.63 (0.43–0.92)
Hip fracture	0.75 (0.68–0.84)	0.66 (0.45–0.98)
Stroke	0.45 (1.10–1.92)	1.41 (1.07–1.85)
Pulmonary embolism	2.1 (1.2–3.8)	2.13 (1.39–3.25)
Coronary artery disease	0.61 (0.45–0.82)	1.29 (1.02–1.63)

Reprinted from Grodstein et al. (31), with permission.
[a]References (25,26,28–30,32).
[b]Reference (31).

LESSONS LEARNED:
SHORTCOMINGS OF OBSERVATIONAL RESEARCH

Observational studies can yield either smaller or larger risk estimates compared with randomized trials. However, observational data tend to underestimate harm. As a result, those that do identify a signal for harm can be useful as hypothesis-generating studies that have implications for safety surveillance. Many observational cohort studies have benefited from a long period of surveillance, such as the Nurses' Health Study, but few are designed to capture clinical events early during therapy. In the Nurses' Health Study, information was collected at 2-year intervals, a study design that could not identify women who both initiated HRT and had an acute MI within a 2-year period (26). Such women were considered nonusers of HRT, leading to overestimation of the rate of CAD in healthy women and ultimately a false conclusion about the cardioprotective benefits of HRT.

Several other biases can be inherent in observational study designs. Studies such as the Nurses' Health Study are prone to selection bias when subjects are lost to follow-up. Classification bias can occur when personnel responsible for data collection know the status of each subject. In the case of HRT, indication bias further confounded the study. Until the mid-1990s, HRT was contraindicated in women with hypertension, diabetes, and cardiovascular disease. Thus, HRT users historically were healthier, were more educated, were of a higher socioeconomic status, and had fewer cardiovascular risk factors. Blinded randomization in trials can preclude such biases and minimize the confounding caused by residual differences between cohorts.

SUMMARY AND FUTURE DIRECTIONS IN OBSERVATIONAL RESEARCH

Current trends are placing a greater importance on the appropriate use of observational data. First, technology is enabling the rapid acquisition of real-world clinical data, which can then be used for observational analyses. Electronic health records are facilitating surveillance of the efficacy and risks of established and emerging therapies. The US Food and Drug Administration, for example, is piloting an active safety surveillance system called Mini-Sentinel, which can actively monitor approved medical products using electronic health information from more than 60 million people (34).

Second, observational analyses of such real-world data will also play an important role in understanding therapeutic risks and benefits through direct comparisons of treatment options. To date, many randomized trials are studies of efficacy rather than effectiveness relative to alternative options. In outlining the national priorities for comparative effectiveness research, the Institute of Medicine has articulated the need to improve the quality of health care through not only the pragmatic design of randomized trials but also the judicious use of observational data (35). Proper recognition biases and unmeasured confounding can allow observational data to provide the best understanding of treatment options when trials are not possible.

Third, when trials *are* possible, observational analyses of electronic health information can be used to accelerate clinical discovery and spur future trials. Studies conducted within online communities using matching algorithms are emerging as another means of monitoring the safety and effectiveness of therapies (36). This merging of randomized trials with the environment of online communities and registries emphasizes the continuing need to learn from prior observational studies to improve the future of clinical research.

REFERENCES

1. Lloyd-Jones D, et al. Executive summary: heart disease and stroke statistics–2010 update: a report from the American Heart Association. *Circulation*. 2010;121(7):948-954.
2. Tricoci P, Allen JM, Kramer JM, Califf RM, Smith SC Jr. Scientific evidence underlying the ACC/AHA clinical practice guidelines. *JAMA*. 2009;301(8): 831-841.
3. Singh M, et al. Trends in the association between age and in-hospital mortality after percutaneous coronary intervention: National Cardiovascular Data Registry experience. *Circ Cardiovasc Interv*. 2009;2(1):20-26.
4. Bauer T, et al. Predictors of hospital mortality in the elderly undergoing percutaneous coronary intervention for acute coronary syndromes and stable angina. *Int J Cardiol*. 2011;151(2):164-169.
5. Lee PY, Alexander KP, Hammill BG, Pasquali SK, Peterson ED. Representation of elderly persons and women in published randomized trials of acute coronary syndromes. *JAMA*. 2001;286(6):708-713.
6. Alexander KP, et al. Acute coronary care in the elderly, part I: Non-ST-segment-elevation acute coronary syndromes: a scientific statement for healthcare professionals from the American Heart Association Council on Clinical Cardiology: in collaboration with the Society of Geriatric Cardiology. *Circulation*. 2007;115(19):2549-2569.
7. GRACE Investigators. Rationale and design of the GRACE (Global Registry of Acute Coronary Events) Project: a multinational registry of patients hospitalized with acute coronary syndromes. *Am Heart J*. 2001;141(2):190-199.
8. Hoekstra JW, et al. Improving the care of patients with non-ST-elevation acute coronary syndromes in the emergency department: the CRUSADE initiative. *Acad Emerg Med*. 2002;9(11):1146-1155.
9. Metz BK, et al. Randomized comparison of direct thrombin inhibition versus heparin in conjunction with fibrinolytic therapy for acute myocardial infarction: results from the GUSTO-IIb trial. Global use of strategies to open occluded coronary arteries in acute coronary syndromes (GUSTO-IIb) investigators. *J Am Coll Cardiol*. 1998;31(7):1493-1498.
10. The PARAGON Investigators. International, randomized, controlled trial of lamifiban (a platelet glycoprotein IIb/IIIa inhibitor), heparin, or both in unstable angina. *Circulation*. 1998;97(24):2386-2395.
11. Mukherjee D, et al. Promise of combined low-molecular-weight heparin and platelet glycoprotein IIb/IIIa inhibition: results from Platelet IIb/IIIa Antagonist for the Reduction of Acute coronary syndrome events in a Global Organization Network B (PARAGON B). *Am Heart J*. 2002;144(6): 995-1002.

12. The PURSUIT Trial Investigators. Inhibition of platelet glycoprotein IIb/IIIa with eptifibatide in patients with acute coronary syndromes. *N Engl J Med.* 1998;339(7):436-443.

13. Simoons ML. Effect of glycoprotein IIb/IIIa receptor blocker abciximab on outcome in patients with acute coronary syndromes without early coronary revascularisation: the GUSTO IV-ACS randomised trial. *Lancet.* 2001;357 (9272):1915-1924.

14. Homocysteine Studies Collaboration. Homocysteine and risk of ischemic heart disease and stroke: a meta-analysis. *JAMA.* 2002;288(16):2015-2022.

15. Arnesen H, et al. Sustained prothrombotic profile after hip replacement surgery: the influence of prolonged prophylaxis with dalteparin. *J Thromb Haemost.* 2003;1(5):97-15.

16. Nygård O, et al. Plasma homocysteine levels and mortality in patients with coronary artery disease. *N Engl J Med.* 1997;337(4):230-236.

17. Boushey CJ, Beresford SA, Omenn GS, Motulsky AG. A quantitative assessment of plasma homocysteine as a risk factor for vascular disease. Probable benefits of increasing folic acid intakes. *JAMA.* 1995;274(13): 1049-1057.

18. Wald DS, Law M, Morris JK. Homocysteine and cardiovascular disease: evidence on causality from a meta-analysis. *BMJ.* 2002;325(7374):1202.

19. Lonn E, et al. Homocysteine lowering with folic acid and B vitamins in vascular disease. *N Engl J Med.* 2006;354(15):1567-1577.

20. Bønaa KH, et al. Homocysteine lowering and cardiovascular events after acute myocardial infarction. *N Engl J Med.* 2006;354(15):1578-1588.

21. Stampfer MJ, et al. Vitamin E consumption and the risk of coronary disease in women. *N Engl J Med.* 1993;328(20):1444-1449.

22. Rimm EB, et al. Vitamin E consumption and the risk of coronary heart disease in men. *N Engl J Med.* 1993;328(20):1450-1456.

23. Hodis HN, et al. Serial coronary angiographic evidence that antioxidant vitamin intake reduces progression of coronary artery atherosclerosis. *JAMA.* 1995;273(23):1849-1854.

24. Yusuf S, Dagenais G, Pogue J, Bosch J, Sleight P. Vitamin E supplementation and cardiovascular events in high-risk patients. The Heart Outcomes Prevention Evaluation Study Investigators. *N Engl J Med.* 2000;342(3):154-160.

25. Grady D, et al. Hormone therapy to prevent disease and prolong life in postmenopausal women. *Ann Intern Med.* 1992;117(12):1016-1037.

26. Grodstein F, et al. A prospective, observational study of postmenopausal hormone therapy and primary prevention of cardiovascular disease. *Ann Intern Med.* 2000;133(12):933-941.

27. Rossouw JE, et al. Risks and benefits of estrogen plus progestin in healthy postmenopausal women: principal results From the Women's Health Initiative randomized controlled trial. *JAMA.* 2002;288(3):321-333.

28. Grodstein F, Newcomb PA, Stampfer MJ. Postmenopausal hormone therapy and the risk of colorectal cancer: a review and meta-analysis. *Am J Med.* 1999;106(5):574-582.

29. Grodstein F, et al. Prospective study of exogenous hormones and risk of pulmonary embolism in women. *Lancet.* 1996;348(9033):983-987.

30. Grodstein F, Stampfer MJ. The epidemiology of postmenopausal hormone therapy and cardiovascular disease. In: *Goldhaber SZ, Ridker PM, eds. Thrombosis and Thromboembolism.* New York: Marcel Dekker; 2002.

31. Grodstein F, Clarkson TB, Manson JE. Understanding the divergent data on postmenopausal hormone therapy. *N Engl J Med.* 2003;348(7):645-650.

32. Marchioli R, et al. Early protection against sudden death by n-3 polyunsaturated fatty acids after myocardial infarction: time-course analysis of the results of the Gruppo Italiano per lo Studio della Sopravvivenza nell'Infarto Miocardico (GISSI)-Prevenzione. *Circulation.* 2002;105(16):1897-1903.

33. Cline JM, et al. Effects of hormone replacement therapy on the mammary gland of surgically postmenopausal cynomolgus macaques. *Am J Obstet Gynecol.* 1996;174(1 Pt 1):93-100.

34. Behrman RE, et al. Developing the Sentinel System—a national resource for evidence development. *N Engl J Med.* 2011;364(6):498-499.

35. Committee on Comparative Effectiveness Research Prioritization, Institute of Medicine. *Initial National Priorities for Comparative Effectiveness Research.* Washington DC: National Academies Press; 2009.

36. Wicks P, Vaughan TE, Massagli MP, Heywood J. Accelerated clinical discovery using self-reported patient data collected online and a patient-matching algorithm. *Nat Biotechnol.* 2011;29(5):411-414.

Index

Note: Page numbers followed "*f*" denote figures; those followed by "*t*" denote tables.